'MERCIFUL RELEASE'

MANCHESTER
UNIVERSITY PRESS

'Merciful release'

The history of the British euthanasia movement

N. D. A. Kemp

MANCHESTER UNIVERSITY PRESS
Manchester and New York

distributed exclusively in the USA by Palgrave

Published by Manchester University Press
Oxford Road, Manchester M13 9NR, UK
and Room 400, 175 Fifth Avenue, New York, NY 10010, USA
www.manchesteruniversitypress.co.uk

Distributed exclusively in the USA by
Palgrave, 175 Fifth Avenue, New York,
NY 10010, USA

Distributed exclusively in Canada by
UBC Press, University of British Columbia, 2029 West Mall,
Vancouver, BC, Canada V6T 1Z2

British Library Cataloguing-in-Publication Data
A catalogue record for this book is available from the British Library

Library of Congress Cataloging-in-Publication Data applied for

ISBN 0 7190 6123 7 *hardback*
    0 7190 6124 5 *paperback*

First published 2002

10 09 08 07 06 05 04 03 02   10 9 8 7 6 5 4 3 2 1

Typeset in Palatino with Frutiger
by Action Publishing Technology Limited, Gloucester
Printed in Great Britain
by Bell & Bain Ltd, Glasgow

Contents

List of figures and tables

Figures

Tables

Acknowledgements

This book could not have been written without the help of a large number of people. I would like to thank Professor Michael Burleigh who first stimulated my interest in euthanasia and eugenics while at the London School of Economics. This initial enthusiasm was channelled effectively thanks to the help and encouragement of Professor Brian Harrison, Professor Paul Weindling, Professor Jane Lewis and Dr Martin Conway, all at the University of Oxford. I would also like to thank Alison Whittle of Manchester University Press who decided to commission this work.

My research was facilitated by a grant from the British Academy, for which I am extremely grateful. I am similarly grateful to the staffs of: the Bodleian Library; the Radcliffe Science Library; the Wellcome Institute; the Contemporary Medical Archives Centre; the Wellcome Unit for the History of Medicine, Oxford; the Public Record Office; the Galton Institute; the British Humanist Society; the British Medical Association; and the British Library of Political and Economic Science. The Voluntary Euthanasia Society was particularly generous in its assistance by granting me permission to reproduce photographs from its archive.

I owe an enormous debt of gratitude to all at Balliol College, Oxford, past and present, who provided me with such a congenial environment in which to work and relax. I must pay special thanks to my family and friends who sustained me throughout, and in particular to Constance.

Introduction

Socio-medical issues have become an increasingly popular area of research for historians. There is now a profusion of literature examining the histories of birth control,[1] abortion,[2] infanticide[3] and eugenics.[4] In part this has been prompted by a natural curiosity to see how past eras have treated issues which remain contentious today. The subject of euthanasia currently enjoys a great deal of media attention[5] and is a storm centre of medical, philosophical and legal debate. Yet with the exception of the Nazi 'euthanasia' programme,[6] it has received comparatively little attention from historians.[7] This is perhaps a little surprising. As H. G. Wells remarked, 'Under scientific analysis the essential facts of life are clearly shown to be two – birth and death.'[8] Because death is inevitable, euthanasia is potentially of interest to everyone. Furthermore, developments in medical technology have made questions of the primacy of quality or quantity of life particularly pertinent. This is reflected by the large amount of bio-ethical literature which now exists.[9] Despite such contemporary interest, and despite the fact that it was in Britain that the first euthanasia movement was pioneered, this study provides the only comprehensive analysis of the British euthanasia movement. It begins by examining the inception of the modern euthanasia debate in 1870 and traces the evolution of the movement and debate until the defeat of the second Voluntary Euthanasia Bill in 1969. Explanations for the persistent prohibition of euthanasia and developments in the discourse from 1969 to the present day are explored in a concluding chapter.

At the outset we should attempt to clarify precisely what we mean by 'euthanasia', for although the term is commonplace it is also complex. In modern discourse euthanasia tends to be understood as a voluntary death assisted by a physician. The typical scenario is that of a patient suffering from a terminal illness afflicted by acute pain and suffering who asks his physician either to provide or administer a lethal dose of narcotics in order to secure a premature death.

But the term has also been used in connection with the killing of mentally incompetent patients; for example patients in a persistent vegetative state who have no prospect of regaining the capacity for rational existence, but who function physically with the aid of intravenous feeding or artificial respiration. Cases of this nature are essentially a product of twentieth-century medical technological advance. They have muddied the boundaries between life and death, complicating the moral questions endemic to medical decision making. These developments have also given rise to the concept of the living will or advance directive. This is a document in which an individual makes known his or her wish that should they fall prey to a life-threatening condition accompanied by an inability to make rational decisions they would prefer to receive no further medical treatment. The advance directive enables a patient to register his or her wish to die a premature death rather than a lingering one. This form of euthanasia remains voluntary in the sense that the patient has registered his wishes while *compos mentis*. In other cases, a patient may nominate a friend or relative to make important decisions regarding the desirability of particular forms of treatment in the event of their mental incapacity. In this case the third party would attempt to act in the patient's best interests by anticipating his or her wishes. Thus even if we separate the notion of euthanasia into voluntary and non-voluntary categories, we have to make further sub-divisions because death may be brought about by either active or passive means. A physician may take the direct action of administering an overdose to his patient and here it is clear that the doctor has killed his patient. But, it is also possible to cause death by withdrawing particular forms of treatment, or by abstaining from treatment which might prolong life. This practice is often referred to as passive euthanasia.

From these examples alone it is clear that the concept of euthanasia is not a monolithic one. Nor does the law regard it as such. Although there remains considerable legal debate, case law has established that particular forms of passive euthanasia are permissible within the framework of the existing law. Advance directives are also considered to be legally binding. But active euthanasia remains outside the boundaries of British law. A physician found to have administered a lethal dose of drugs to a patient with the intention of causing premature death is liable to prosecution for murder. However, if the drugs administered were those commonly used for the relief of pain, it is likely that the physician would avoid prosecution. A side-effect of palliative drugs is that they may also shorten a patient's life as incrementally larger doses are required to deaden the pain. In these circumstances a patient's death may be said to have been an unintended consequence of pain relief. This scenario has been termed the doctrine of double effect. While it is usually raised as a safety net to prevent innocent physicians from wrongful prosecution it provides considerable latitude in the law with regard to euthanasia.

Because of the illicit nature of euthanasia and the concomitant dearth of empirical data this is not a history of the practice of euthanasia. Rather it sets out to clarify the emergence and development of the debates which have accompanied successive attempts to secure endorsement of the various practices which might be grouped under the heading of euthanasia. On numerous occasions cases have come to the attention of the legal authorities and have impinged upon the debate, but they are not in themselves the focus of this study. The book does, however, attempt to explain the legal position on euthanasia and the way in which cases are treated by the judiciary.

To some extent the book can be seen as a new chapter in the history of ideas; it is concerned with debates and arguments. But, it is less philosophically rooted than the majority of literature in that field. Philosophical debate is certainly one aspect of the study, but the history of the movement also requires analysis of theological and legal debates and of the debates which have taken place amongst the medical profession and the broader populace. It draws heavily on the history of medicine and on more mainstream British history. It attempts to link shifts in the euthanasia debate to broader shifts in society, such as the secularisation and liberalisation of values, the impact of evolutionary and eugenic thought, and the impact of the two World Wars. Because it is the first history of its kind a chronological arrangement has been adopted. By establishing precisely what was said when, we avoid assuming that euthanasia debates have a timeless quality. Only after establishing the facts can serious analysis begin. It is also apparent that successive periods each have their own distinctive thematic hue. Put simply the content and context of euthanasia debates has altered markedly from their inception in the 1870s, and over the course of the twentieth century.

In defining euthanasia, we have seen that even in modern discourse, where there is a tendency to think that the term has a very precise meaning, in practice euthanasia can mean several different things. It may refer to suicide by a patient who is gravely ill; requested mercy-killing of a patient by a physician; non-voluntary killing by a physician acting in the best interests of an incompetent patient; and selective non-treatment with the foreseen consequence of a patient's death. Clearly all these forms of euthanasia share a medical dimension, but in accounting for the variety of ways in which the term might be defined, it is instructive to trace its etymology.

The term is a compound of two Greek words 'eu' meaning 'good' and 'thanatos' meaning 'death'. This literal translation of a 'good death', gives some indication that euthanasia has a strong subjective dimension; a 'good death' may be construed in many different ways from different perspectives. Indeed, a central theme of the book is that euthanasia has meant strikingly different things to different people at different times.

Despite its Greek origins, the term appears very infrequently in classical literature. When it does, it refers to a gentle form of death such as that depicted in Suetonius's account of the death of Augustus.[10] It does not denote suicide or mercy-killing by a physician. This immediately brings us to an important methodological issue. Discussion which has employed the term euthanasia has not necessarily been concerned with the deliberate precipitation of death. Similarly, although the word may not have been used at a particular time this need not indicate an absence of discussion about forms of mercy-killing which approximate modern-day concepts of euthanasia.

Classical antiquity provides examples of both cases. While the ethical code of the medical profession as laid down in the Hippocratic Oath explicitly prohibited physician-assisted suicide, stating 'I will neither give a deadly drug to anybody if asked for it, nor will I make a suggestion to this effect'[11] this has actually been interpreted as proof that abstention from the practice was not universal. '[I]f the question had not arisen, it would not have occurred to anyone to codify the prohibition.'[12] Yet to suggest that '[t]his form of "euthanasia" was an everyday reality',[13] as Ludwig Edelstein has done, is perhaps a little misleading. Edelstein has transposed a modern definition of euthanasia onto a period when, as we have seen, the term meant something rather different. Nevertheless, it is clear that the notion of justifiable suicide enjoyed considerable support in ancient Greece. This is not to suggest that suicide was subject to unequivocal approval in classical antiquity. Pythagoras writing in the sixth century BC believed man to be the chattel of God and his life was not to be ended without God's command.[14] Plato suggested that as the soldier of God man must stay at his post until called,[15] and Aristotle rejected suicide on the grounds that man owed a duty to the state.[16] Yet for all three suicide was acceptable in cases of incurable disease; Aristotle and Pliny even alluded to the particular diseases which were regarded as providing sufficient justification for a voluntary death.[17] The Stoics also took a sympathetic stance towards suicide. Zeno the founder of the school was said to have committed suicide after wrenching his finger.

If we can establish that physician-assisted suicide, and suicide in the specific circumstances of incurable or painful disease were discussed and practised in the classical world, then it is necessary to explain why this history of the euthanasia movement should begin in 1870. The explanation is certainly not one of language alone. It is true there was nothing which was sufficiently concerted to be called a movement before the 1870s, or perhaps before the 1930s when the Voluntary Euthanasia Legalisation Society was founded. But it is also important to highlight the factors which precluded discussion of euthanasia so that we can then identify the catalysts for the emergence of a euthanasia movement.

Following the Roman conquest of Greece, the Stoic philosophy concerning suicide was widely endorsed.[18] This sympathetic view seems to have remained in force until some two hundred years after the death of Christ. Thereafter the circumstances in which suicide was considered legitimate were progressively restricted. Many of the patristic writers had condoned suicide in exceptional circumstances, notably in defence of chastity or in order to achieve martyrdom but not in cases of painful and incurable illness. Lactantius suggested that it was 'wicked to bring death upon oneself voluntarily, unless one was "expecting all torture and death" at the hands of the pagan persecutors'.[19] St Jerome permitted suicide only in defence of chastity.[20] But, ultimately complete prohibition was advocated. St Augustine argued 'with fine simplicity that the Scriptures nowhere authorized us to eliminate ourselves'.[21] Suicide was regarded as a cowardly act, and the 'Church followed Augustine's view that true heroism consisted in suffering as a soldier of Christ in preference to killing oneself'.[22] Suicide in all circumstances was deemed to be contrary to natural law. In the course of the fifth century Church Law codified this view when the Council of Arles denounced suicide as 'diabolically inspired'.[23] This resolute position was reinforced in the thirteenth century when St Thomas Aquinas declared suicide to be the most fatal of sins because it could not be repented of.[24] As early as AD 563 Christian burial was denied to suicides.[25] The rigid Christian view of the sanctity of human life effectively precluded any form of suicide.

This inflexible Christian position remained largely unaltered throughout the medieval period. But during the Renaissance there appears to have been a slight thawing of ideas. In the second book of *Utopia* (1516), Sir Thomas More counselled suicide for patients afflicted with painful and incurable diseases. In Europe as a whole, intellectual interest in suicide had begun to increase by the early seventeenth century. This seems to have been prompted by 'religious persecution and war' which gave rise to such questions as whether zealots and martyrs were 'guilty of sin if they had in some sense killed themselves? Might a virgin kill herself to preserve her chastity? ... Might a patriot seek certain death for his country?'[26]

In the course of the seventeenth century, discussion about suicide became even more frequent. In 1648, in a book entitled *Biathanatos*, the Anglican priest, poet and dean of St Paul's, John Donne, arguing from a Christian perspective declared that suicide was not inherently evil.[27] He argued that the act was not always prompted by desperation, but could on occasion indicate consideration and courage.[28]

By the following century suicide had become the subject of considerable intellectual debate. '[I]n the age of reason opponents rose in public to argue that suicide might be a guiltless action.'[29] The view of the libertine was that individual judgement was a 'legitimate indication of the will of divine Providence'.[30] Arguments which had urged against suicide such as an individual's civic obligations were modified to highlight an individual's civic rights. The most notable philosophical contribution to this debate, was David Hume's essay *On Suicide* published in 1777. Hume considered man to have a 'native liberty' in particular circumstances, notably pain and disease, to effect death at the time of his own choosing. Exactly what led Hume to the subject is not clear, but it does seem that suicide was 'one of the serious public questions of his time'.[31] On empirical grounds he sought to show that suicide might 'be free from every imputation of guilt or blame'. Hume's argument was especially pertinent to medical ethics. He noted, for example, that medical science was already interfering with Divine Providence through its efforts to prolong life and if this was acceptable, then the shortening of life was similarly legitimate. Such arguments served as an important precursor to the euthanasia debate.

In 1790 the Reverend Charles Moore while condemning suicide suggested that the 'most excusable cause' seemed to be an 'emaciated body; when a man labours under the tortures of an incurable disorder, and seems to live only to be a burden to himself and his friends. This was thought to be a sufficient apology for the action in ancient days and can only be combated in modern ones by the force and energy of that true religion, which both points out the duty and the reward of implicit resignation.'[32] Although particular authors were advancing a more sympathetic view of justifiable suicide the modern 'euthanasia' debate had not yet commenced.[33]

Discussion regarding justifiable suicide certainly took place, but the term, 'euthanasia' was not used in this context. In the early seventeenth century Francis Bacon had plucked the term from relative obscurity and used it in a medical context. He had suggested that the duty of the physician included not only the restoration of health but also the mitigation of pain and dolours 'and not only when such mitigation may conduce to recovery, but when it may serve a fair and easy passage'.[34] Yet, while he had indicated that the physician should play a more active role in easing the dying moments of his suffering patient, this did not include deliberately precipitating death. Thus the term retained its classical meaning, albeit with the physician now at the centre of the picture. Bacon's use of the term in this new sense seems to have been completely isolated.

During the nineteenth century in addition to its classical meaning of a good, gentle or happy death the term 'euthanasia' had strong religious associations. Surveying the literature of this period one finds titles including *Euthanasia; Or The State of Man After Death*[35] and *Euthanasia, Sermons and Poems, In Memory of Departed Friends*.[36] In the hands of pious Christians 'euthanasia' was concerned with issues such as the immortality of the soul and certainly not the deliberate precipitation of death. The Evangelical revival of the late eighteenth and the first half of the nineteenth century affirmed a strongly theological notion of 'euthanasia'. This notion of the 'good death' drew heavily on the large body of devotional literature known as the *'ars moriendi*, the art of dying' which had emerged in the late medieval and early modern periods.[37] Ideally death would take place in the home surrounded by one's family; the presence of a doctor was not typical.[38] A lengthy illness was to be welcomed because it provided the dying person with sufficient time to complete his spiritual and temporal business before death. The patient should be lucid until the end so that he might seek forgiveness, bear suffering with fortitude and demonstrate that he was worthy of salvation. 'The state of the individual's soul at the moment of death was deemed of vital importance, since there was an immediate divine judgement on each individual at death, making constant preparation essential.'[39] Sudden death was considered to be highly unfortunate because it offered no opportunity for spiritual preparation or repentance and thus the prospect of eternal hell-fire loomed. Suicide was regarded as the worst form of death. Modern-day notions of 'euthanasia' and those of the Victorian Evangelical were clearly not the same.

Towards the end of the nineteenth century, however, the religious notion of the 'good death' seems to have waned as the Evangelical movement itself began to decline. 'Family accounts of deathbed scenes' from the 1870s onwards are said to have 'lacked the intense piety and spiritual fervour of earlier decades'.[40] Preoccupation with spiritual well-being appears to have been gradually eclipsed by the desire to die in the absence of physical pain and suffering. This time frame coincides very closely with the appearance of the first text to use the term 'euthanasia' in the modern sense of physician-assisted suicide. Only at this time can we say that the 'euthanasia' debate really began. This was the first intersection of the debate about justifiable self-murder and a redefinition of the term 'euthanasia'. This intersection provides the starting point for the book.

Notes

1   Richard Soloway, *Demography and Degeneration: Eugenics and the Declining Birthrate in Twentieth-Century Britain* (London, 1990).
2   Barbara Brookes, *Abortion in Britain* 1900–1967 (London, 1988).
3   Mark Jackson, *New-born Child Murder: Women, Illegitimacy and the Courts in Eighteenth-Century England* (Manchester, 1996).
4   Daniel Kevles, *In the Name of Eugenics* (New York, 1985).
5   See for example *The Times*, 6 Jan. 1999, p. 1.
6   Michael Burleigh, *Death and Deliverance: 'Euthanasia' in Germany 1900–1945* (Cambridge, 1994); Henry Friedlander, *The Origins of Nazi Genocide: From Euthanasia To The Final Solution* (London, 1995); Paul Weindling, *Health, Race and German Politics Between National Unification and Nazism 1870–1945* (Cambridge, 1989).
7   W. Bruce Fye, 'Active euthanasia: an historical survey of its conceptual origins and introduction into medical thought', *Bulletin of the History of Medicine*, 1968, pp. 493–502; I. Van Der Sluis, 'The movement for euthanasia 1875–1975', *Janus*, Vol. 66, pp. 131–72; Ezekiel J. Emanuel, 'The history of euthanasia debates in the United States and Britain', *Annals of Internal Medicine*, 15 Nov. 1994, Vol. 121, No. 10, pp. 793–802; Ranaan Gillon, 'Suicide and voluntary euthanasia: historical perspective', in A. B. Downing (ed.), *Euthanasia and the Right to Die* (London, 1969).
8   H. G. Wells, *Anticipations* (London, 1902) p. 297.
9   See for example: Peter Singer, *Rethinking Life and Death* (Oxford, 1994); Marvin Kohl (ed.), *Beneficent Euthanasia* (New York, 1975); Ronald Dworkin, *Life's Dominion* (London, 1993).
10 *Suetonius I*, translated by J. C. Rolfe (Cambridge, Mass [1913], 1989), p. 281.
11 Hippocratic Oath (Edelstein translation), L. Edelstein, 'The Hippocratic oath', *Supplement to the Bulletin of the History of Medicine*, No. 1 (Baltimore, 1943).
12 Danielle Gourevitch, 'Suicide among the sick in classical antiquity', *Bulletin of the History of Medicine*, 1969, 43, p. 505.
13 Edelstein, *The Hippocratic Oath*, p. 10.
14 De Senectude: 72 Cicero, in John Burnett, *Early Greek Philosophy* (London, 1892) p. 108. [cf. Cicero, *Cato Major* 20 (72 sq.) and *De Officiis*, i. 31 (112)].
15 *Laws* IX, 873.
16 These examples are cited in Ranaan Gillon, 'Suicide and voluntary euthanasia', pp. 173–92. [Aristotle, *Politics*, 1335b, 19ff.].
17 See Edelstein, *The Hippocratic Oath*, p. 9, note 9.
18 Gillon, 'Suicide and voluntary euthanasia', p. 175.
19 *Divine institutiones*, vi. 17, cited in Joseph Fletcher, *Morals and Medicine* (Princeton, 1955) p. 177.
20 *Commentarii in Jonam*, i. 12, cited in *Ibid*.
21 *De civitate dei*, i. 16 sq., cited in Fletcher, pp. 178–9.
22 S. E. Sprott, *The English Debate on Suicide from Donne to Hume* (Illinois, 1961) p. 6.
23 Gillon, 'Suicide and voluntary euthanasia', p. 177.
24 *Summa Theologica*, ii. –ii 64.5.3.
25 Edward Westermarck, *Christianity and Morals* (London, 1939) p. 254.
26 Sprott, *The English Debate*, pp. 16–17.

27 John Donne, *Biathanatos* (London, 1648) p. 179.

28 Cyrett, *The English Debate* p. 20.

29 *Ibid.*, p. 94.

30 *Ibid.*, p. 98.

31 *Ibid.*, p. 128.

32 Charles Moore, *A Full Inquiry into the Subject of Suicide* (London, 1790) p. 270.

33 For a fuller discussion of attitudes to suicide in the early modern period see Michael MacDonald and Terence R. Murphy, *Sleepless Souls* (Oxford, 1990).

34 Francis Bacon, *New Atlantis* (Oxford, 1924) cited in Ezekiel Emanuel, 'The history of euthanasia debates in the United States and Britain', p. 794.

35 Revd Luke Booker, *Euthanasia; Or The State Of Man After Death* (London, 1822).

36 Revd George Cole, *Euthanasia, Sermons And Poems, In Memory of Departed Friends* (London, 1868).

37 Pat Jalland, *Death in the Victorian Family* (Oxford, 1996) p. 19.

38 *Ibid.*, p. 26.

39 *Ibid.*, p. 17.

40 *Ibid.*, p. 51.

1

The 'euthanasia' debate of the 1870s: the controversy launched

The origins of the modern euthanasia debate can be traced to a brief but concerted debate which took place among a small number of participants during the early 1870s. This chapter offers explanations for the emergence of this discussion and maps the contours of the debate.

In contrast to the euthanasia debate of the late twentieth century this was essentially a philosophical enterprise in which the medical profession played no part. The debate was tied inextricably to a number of objections to the Christian doctrine of the sanctity of human life; some of which were novel, some not. These objections elicited alternative sets of ethical criteria upon which the worth of human life might be determined. As a result a multiplicity of different arguments in favour of different types of euthanasia were advanced. It is suggested that the plurality of conceptions of 'worthwhile life' which were so manifest in this debate have been responsible for the persistent ambiguity with which the term 'euthanasia' has been shrouded. By defining worthwhile life in different ways, different authors advocated euthanasia for several groups of people. Thus we find that different authors used the term euthanasia to advocate the voluntary killing of terminally ill patients, patients afflicted with severe pain, but also individuals whose ailments made them a burden to the community; this including the proposal of non-voluntary killing of mental defectives. The resulting ambiguity surrounding the term euthanasia has ensured sustained opposition to the practice. The elucidation of these themes will provide a constant point of reference throughout the book.

The spark of the debate is to be located in a volume of diverse essays[1] published in 1870 entitled *Essays of the Birmingham*

Speculative Club.[2] With no coherent theme this collection was produced by the individual members of a small club which over the course of a number of years had met periodically to discuss social and philosophical issues. None of the authors were professional philosophers, rather they were all amateurs 'engaged in the daily pursuit of their respective trades or professions'.[3] Nor were the essays the collective product of the society. Although the circulation of this rather obscure volume was small, it was brought to the attention of a much larger audience by the scholarly periodicals which were enjoying their heyday during the 1870s. The reform and expansion of the universities had begun to provide a new calibre of reader and contributor.[4] This combined with the abolition of stamp tax had provided an ideal environment for such literature to flourish. As Kent suggests, 'Higher journalism, the journalism of the more dignified organs of opinion, the reviews, the superior magazines ... was one of the most characteristic cultural manifestations of nineteenth-century Britain.'[5] This was the arena in which the first 'euthanasia' debate thrived.

The *Essays* were first reviewed in *The Saturday Review,*[6] a journal which 'offered serious and well-informed judgement in a tone of deliberately hard-headed detachment'.[7] It suggested that the most 'remarkable' of the essays was that written by a school teacher[8] named Samuel D. Williams jun. entitled 'Euthanasia'.[9] This was an eloquent and forceful argument in favour of physician-assisted suicide which served to redefine the term 'euthanasia', divorcing it from the passive connotations with which it had been associated since classical antiquity, and imbuing it with the notion of justifiable mercy-killing. Williams's essay effectively introduced this ethical conundrum into popular discourse, and was responsible for defining many of the parameters of the ensuing debate. Its significance is such that it deserves to be rehearsed in some detail.

The purpose of Williams's essay was to demonstrate the 'reasonableness' of the following proposition:

> That in all cases of hopeless and painful illness, it should be the recognized duty of the medical attendant, whenever so desired by the patient, to administer chloroform or such other anaesthetic as may by-and-bye supersede chloroform – so as to destroy consciousness at once, and put the sufferer to a quick and painless death; all needful precautions being adopted to prevent any possible abuse

of such duty; and means being taken to establish, beyond the possibility of doubt or question, that the remedy was applied at the express wish of the patient.[10]

Within the space of three years the essay was already on its fourth reprint. The preface to this edition remarked that euthanasia was a subject which should not be ignored, it had prompted 'some of the finest reflections of Seneca', and was supported by that great man and emperor, Marcus Aurelius, who had allegedly shortened his life by refusing sustenance during his final illness. If the subject had so engaged such great historic figures it was certainly worth a 'passing thought from us "giddy moderns"'.[11] Even Sir Thomas More, a devout Christian, in a work entitled *Utopia* written over three hundred years ago had 'advocated what the author of "Euthanasia" does, neither more nor less'.[12]

Williams's argument was certainly eloquent, but it was – as this preface recognised – essentially a discussion of the ethics of suicide for the terminally ill and those experiencing extreme suffering; an ethical issue which had engaged the Stoics over a thousand years ago.[13] Of course it is possible that Williams's essay was simply the product of an abstract philosophical reflection upon an age-old issue, but it seems likely that there were a number of more tangible factors which may explain the emergence of such discussion at this time.

Although this was a debate which neither originated from nor engaged the medical profession, medical innovations did provide a considerable catalyst for the discussion of ethical questions pertaining to life and death. Indeed, while only a handful of papers have examined the history of the euthanasia movement in Britain, all have noted the importance of developments in analgesia and anaesthesia.[14] This seems entirely justified. The nineteenth century had seen enormous advances in this field. In 1816 Frederick Setürner a German apothecary's assistant had succeeded in isolating morphine from opium, and in 1855 Alexander Wood had developed the hypodermic syringe, facilitating the direct introduction of morphine into the bloodstream rather than the more protracted method via the digestive system. The 1840s had also seen the development of ether as a surgical anaesthetic which had been popularised in Britain by Robert Liston and which was subsequently superseded by chloroform due to its ease of administration.

As Samuel Williams recognised, innovations of this nature exposed medical ethics to notable pressures. The use of chloroform had initially been opposed in the strongest terms, particularly from religious quarters. Efforts to escape pain were interpreted as 'evidence of impatience with the ways of Providence and symptoms of revolt against the decree "In sorrow shalt thou bring forth;" ... they ... were not sparing in their prophecies of evil to come on those who practised, and those who submitted to, the innovation they denounced.'[15] Despite such early objection the practice was soon subject to almost universal approval. In 1847 James Young Simpson, an Edinburgh physician, had used chloroform for the relief of pain during childbirth and the practice was given a further boost when Queen Victoria gave birth under its influence. According to Williams the discovery of chloroform as an anaesthetic was '[o]ne of the very greatest practical benefits which science has hitherto conferred on mankind'.[16] The employment of anaesthetics to ease entry into life and for the purpose of surgical operations was increasingly deemed ethical and commonplace. The patient about to be operated on was thus provided with 'a refuge from conscious suffering'.[17] But the dying man 'about to suffer at the hand of nature' whose armoury was deemed to be 'terribly great' was left prostrate, bereft of 'hope of help'. This prompted the enquiry of why the inhaler should 'not be seen as unfailingly by the bed of death, as it is on the operating table'?[18]

Having alluded to this apparent anomaly in man's ethical outlook it was suggested that in all cases of painful and terminal illness, the medical attendant should be *obliged* to administer an anaesthetic in order to avoid the 'last worst pang that poor human nature has to undergo' due to the 'temporary paroxysms of a violent and dangerous illness'.[19] In fact Williams was not the first to have advocated such a measure. As early as 1856 Joseph Bullar, a medical man, had noted the effectiveness of opium in promoting 'euthanasia'[20] in terminal phthisis.[21] In 1866 Bullar also advocated the use of chloroform for the alleviation of pain and suffering in the dying patient. Significantly, he noted that he 'felt nervously anxious at first of giving her too much'.[22] Moreover, he observed that the inhalation of chloroform served to prolong life, it raised the pulse and respiration became 'slower and more natural. ... it seemed to act like the tonic stimulus of food or wine in stronger bodily condition, and at a time when neither of these could be given'.[23] His use of the term was thus classical. Williams on the other hand argued that the patient's consciousness should be promptly and irrevocably extinguished in order to secure a quick and painless death.

The publicity which the *Saturday Review* had provided ensured that other writers would engage with this issue. The Victorian periodicals were after all a commercial venture. As well as providing a forum for the discussion of such issues the periodical was a tool for creating controversy and euthanasia was nothing if not controversial; it was the ideal mechanism for boosting sales. An editorial in *The Spectator* offered the first response in what was to become a lively debate.[24] Conceding that Williams's argument was forcible, it was rejected on practical and religious grounds. It claimed that euthanasia would place an 'intolerable' responsibility upon the patient, his physician and friends. The sick man 'his temper irritated, his will enfeebled by suffering' would be placed in the position of having to make a decision of 'supreme' and 'irrevocable' importance, and the physician would be 'degraded' from 'healer' to 'executioner'. He would be called upon 'to renounce the noblest aspiration of his art, which at least proposes to itself the ideal of a power which no disease shall resist. When is he to say "This malady is incurable"?'[25] Not only was 'euthanasia' contrary to the Hippocratic Oath, perhaps more importantly it was contrary to Judeo-Christian teaching which stressed the sanctity of human life. It was this which had ensured the persistent prohibition of such practices in the western world.

According to Genesis, man had been created in the image of God. God had also given him dominion 'over the fish of the sea, and over the fowl of the air, and over the earth, and over every creeping thing that creepeth upon earth'.[26] To this had been added the notion that man, in contrast to animals, had a soul. To kill a human being was not only to kill an entity created in the image of God, but also to consign that being to its immortal destiny. This was compounded by St Augustine's *Dei Civitate Dei* which had taught that the Biblical injunction, 'Thou shalt not kill', was construed to include self-murder as well as homicide, thus suicide was essentially murder. Furthermore, St Thomas Aquinas, who provided the backbone of Roman Catholic philosophy, regarded it as the worst kind of murder, 'the most grievous thing of all' as it offered no opportunity for repentance, and thereby deliberately denied oneself absolution.

As we noted in the Introduction, the first half of the nineteenth century had been marked by the strong revival of the Evangelical movement with its distinctive notion of the 'good death'. 'Thousands of didactic deathbed scenes in nineteenth-century Evangelical tracts and journals attested to the zeal to save souls by showing people how to die. Death was a primary concern of Evangelical theology, since the doctrines of sin, assurance, and atonement emphasized Christ's sacrifice on the Cross to save people from their sins.'[27] While religious objections certainly provided a considerable obstacle for the advocates of 'euthanasia' the 1870s were a reasonably propitious time at which to enter into such discussion. Without wishing to engage in a tangential discussion about the secularisation of values in nineteenth-century Britain, we might note Owen Chadwick's observation that

> [i]n the years 1860–80 contemporaries were agreed that the tone of society in England was more 'secular'. By that they meant that the atmosphere of middle class conversation; the kind of books which you could find on a drawing-room table, the contents of the magazines to which educated men subscribed whether they were religious or irreligious, the appearance of anti-Christian books on bookstalls at the railway station, the willingness of devout men to meet undevout men in society and to honour them for their sincerity instead of condemning them for their lack of faith.[28]

Notions of the bad death had also begun to change. This was a consequence of the decline of the Evangelical movement and the increasing difficulty which Victorians felt in accepting the idea of a retributive God and the prospect of everlasting torment. This debate had become particularly intense after 1850.[29]

For Williams, man's refusal to curtail terminal suffering was dictated by a number of 'commonplaces' regarding the 'sacredness of life', the 'folly' and 'cowardice' of suicide, the duty of 'submission to the will of GOD' and of 'not quitting one's post, except at the bidding of one's commander,' occasionally accompanied by other commonplaces such as the 'hallowing influences of the sick room, and the beneficent action on the heart of faithful ministration, throughout long and trying illness, to those sick unto death'.[30] He had also made the adroit observation that even among the 'civilized' nations of Europe, the 'sacredness of man's life' tended to be cast aside as soon as political or material interests deemed a recourse to violence necessary. The origins of such arguments are a matter of speculation, but Williams's essay certainly betrayed more than a hint of Humean thinking with regard to its demonstration of the 'hypocrisy' surrounding the sanctity of human life. It is certainly plausible that as a philosophically engaged gentleman Williams was familiar with Hume's essay *On Suicide*.[31] Indeed, the late nineteenth-century debate on 'euthanasia' was in no small part a development of this earlier discussion. The development of anaesthetics provided an additional and novel example of the way in which man interfered with Divine Providence and thus provided a new twist to Hume's ideas. Williams suggested that if you curtail life's duration by a little, 'the same reasoning that justifies a minute's shortening of it, will justify an hour's, a day's, a week's, a month's, a year's; and that all subsequent appeal to the inviolability of life is vain'.[32]

As Ezekiel Emanuel has observed with regard to the euthanasia question in a twentieth-century setting, medical innovations may add to the complexity of ethical questions and the frequency with which they occur, but they are not responsible for the 'creation' of the underlying ethical issues concerning conceptions of worthwhile life.[33]

While suicide was still a criminal offence, attitudes had begun to alter somewhat. The first indication of this was that in 1823 Parliament had repealed the practice of profane burial for suicides. Increasingly suicide was regarded as a symptom of mental illness and this was reflected by the fact that coroner's courts frequently returned verdicts of suicide while of unsound mind which served to reduce the stigma attached to the act. The forfeiture of property which followed suicide was also repealed in 1870. Despite this, there remained forcible opposition to suicide. To advance a watertight argument in favour of suicide as a whole was extremely difficult. As Williams noted there were 'suicides and suicides'.[34] Suicide in the specific circumstances of a painful and terminal illness was thought to be far easier to sustain.

Williams's argument was not without its supporters, the most notable of whom was the Hon. Lionel Arthur Tollemache, rationalist philosopher,[35] Balliol graduate and member of the Athenaeum club.[36] In 1873 Tollemache published a decidedly controversial article entitled 'The Cure for Incurables'[37] in the *Fortnightly Review,* one of the most influential mid-Victorian reviews.[38] Attention was drawn to the fact that many people would have the misfortune of witnessing cancer, creeping paralysis, or some other similarly disturbing condition. Some would also have to endure what was deemed to be 'the hardest fate of all', that of a mortally wounded soldier who desires to die 'but whose wounds are laboriously tended; so that, by an ingenious cruelty, he is kept suffering, against nature, and against his own will'.[39] Confronting the 'theological', 'sentimental' and 'rational'[40] objections to euthanasia Tollemache pointed to apparent inconsistencies in the Church's stance with regard to interference in Divine Providence. According to Christian doctrine pain was to be endured, yet such an argument 'if worth anything' would not only preclude the extinction of pain, but would also prohibit 'its partial mitigation' through the application of opiates. He went on

> as Mr Williams argues, all suffering is represented as the effect of sin, and especially the suffering of childbirth. And the Evangelicals were quite consistent in the opposition that they raised to the use of chloroform in confinements, until fortunately, public opinion became too strong for them. May not their own logic be turned against them, if it should one day appear that the uses of the sedative in childbirth and before death involve the same principle, and must stand and fall together?[41]

Williams had actually argued further, that the ethical distinction which physicians attempted to draw between pain relief and precipitating death was much narrower than often supposed. Pre-empting discussions of the 'doctrine of double effect'[42] he pointed out that a medical attendant who refused to administer a lethal dose to a 'hopelessly suffering' patient, despite being 'implored by him to do so', would usually have no qualms about securing the patient's temporary relief through the administration of opiates or 'other anaesthetics', despite the fact that in so doing he was knowingly shortening the patient's life.[43] Moreover, very few patients, patient's friends or relatives would hesitate in asking the doctor to administer the drug. As he was quick to enquire, if this was so 'what becomes of the sacredness of life?'

Williams's assessment of the matter certainly has considerable appeal. But, in the case cited above we might wish to draw a distinction between the physician's intended and unintended consequences resulting from the application of the pain-killing drug. This is an issue to which we shall return in subsequent chapters.

For Tollemache, man was bound either to 'stretch to the utmost the elastic thread of life' or he was not. If he was so bound then nearly everyone was guilty of 'great wickedness'. If on the other hand there were limits to this duty 'human reason' should be the arbiter and 'human welfare' should be the criterion for judgement. The question of 'euthanasia' should be discussed on social rather than theological grounds.[44] The sanctity of human life is not a concept which admits of degrees. The arguments of Williams and Tollemache purported to demonstrate that in practice the concept was not held to be absolute, if this was so it was a concept which was extremely difficult to sustain. The view that all human life was intrinsically valuable would have to be replaced by an alternative conception of 'worthwhile' life.

Although a number of commentators have made reference to Williams's essay all have tended to underplay the importance of its evolutionary rhetoric. While we should be wary of depicting Darwin as the man responsible for ushering in a secular age[45] we should be similarly cautious of underestimating the importance of evolutionary thought in relation to the questioning of the sanctity of human life. The first half of the nineteenth century was after all a period during which the 'modern outline of the fossil record' had been pieced together, revealing 'the ascent of life from primitive fish and invertebrates through the Age of Reptiles to the Age of Mammals and the world of today'.[46] Indeed, in a notebook entry of 1838 Darwin had remarked that 'Man in his arrogance thinks himself a great work, worthy of the interposition of a deity. More humble and, I believe, true to consider him created from animals'.[47] One does not wish to reduce complex matters to the schoolboy maxim that Darwin 'disproved religion',[48] but if man had evolved from the animals and had not been created in the image of God, the sanctity of human life was clearly problematic.

Indeed, 1870, the date of Williams's publication, is not without significance. Following closely on the heels of *Origin of Species* (1859), and just a year before Darwin's *Descent of Man* (1871), Williams essay was replete with numerous allusions to evolutionary thought. This is perhaps not overly surprising. As Harris notes, '[e]volutionary models and metaphors' became increasingly pervasive in social thought, and by the 1880s 'had become part of the dominant intellectual paradigm of the age.'[49] Not only was evolutionary discourse important with regard to the sanctity of human life, it also provided an air of scientific authority and a host of cutting edge metaphors and 'catch-phrases'[50] upon which to draw. These manifested themselves quite explicitly in the work of the early advocates of 'euthanasia'. Williams, for example, observed that the world was a 'field of mortal struggle' as opposed to a 'beneficent design' whose sole purpose was 'enjoyment'.

> [E]very organised being wages, from the beginning of its career to the end, unceasing war with enemies of all kinds; wherein a universal struggle for mastery, and a universal preying on the weak by the strong is incessant; where conflict, cruelty, suffering, and death are in full activity at every moment in every place, even to the minutest crick or cranny that microscopic existence can occupy; and the only fact in all this scene of carnage that can be pointed to as significant of beneficent design, is the continuous victory of the strong, the continuous crushing out of the weak, and the consequent maintenance of what is called 'the vigour of the race;' the preservation of the hardiest races, and of the hardiest individuals or each race so preserved.[51]

Williams believed that the mitigation of such suffering should be one of man's chief aims in life, he should attempt to bring it within 'bearable proportions.' Human life was at best a 'sorrowful thing' and a 'real alleviation of its pains was the greatest service which man could render to man'.[52] Like all other organisms, the 'natural provision' was for the 'weak to go to the wall'. Employing social Darwinian rhetoric, Williams noted that man already behaved in counter-selective ways. Modern medicine although commendable, effectively sponsored the survival of the 'unfit'. If this was ethically justifiable, then man was similarly justified in preventing the suffering at the end of life which nature saw fit to impose. Man should ensure that the weak went to the wall in the most comfortable fashion.

A desire to minimise the unnecessary and futile suffering at the end of a terminal illness was, and remains the centrepiece of the case for 'euthanasia'. Williams was of the opinion that whenever a man was stricken by disease he was unquestionably right – unless absolutely sure of his ability to endure severe pain – in making full use of the palliatives with which man's genius had furnished him, and 'laying down calmly and deliberately, and painlessly, a life which, but for such palliatives would have to be passed in weary suffering, and closed perhaps in agony'.[53] Indeed, for many it is considered an act of cruelty to prolong a patient's existence when death is both inevitable and imminent, and when the experience is one racked by pain, misery and indignity. The supporters of this view hold that patients should have the autonomy to shape their own conception of when their life is, or is not, 'worthwhile'. Understandably, this would usually take a hedonistic form. A life characterised by acute pain and suffering might reduce 'quality of life' to the extent that the patient deemed his life 'worthless'. The belief that the patient should make his own appraisal of his quality of life was clearly endorsed by Williams. When 'the patient desires to die'[54] his wishes should be respected.

However, during the debate of the 1870s, such arguments were often accompanied by auxiliary ones which lent ambiguity to the concept of 'euthanasia'. 'A transitory thing seldom extending beyond threescore years and ten', life for Williams was difficult to construe in such a way that it was 'sacred', except to the extent that man had a 'duty' to use his life 'nobly' while in possession of it. He suggested that when the possibility of making a noble use of life had evaporated, when life was bereft of use, causing nothing but pain for its possessor, then there could be no violation of the 'sacredness of life, in this sense of the word, when, with the consent of the sufferer, a life is taken away that has ceased to be useful to others, and has become an unbearable infliction to its possessor'.[55]

While we need not question that the sense of being 'an intolerable burden' to oneself was the most important criterion for Williams in deciding whether the application of 'euthanasia' was justified, we must not overlook the first part of this quotation. By invoking such concepts as 'no longer of use to others', we are presented with a further basis on which to assess the justifiability of 'euthanasia'. Indeed, as medical ethicists have suggested, the notion of 'quality of life ... contains at least two distinct meanings that are often unrecognised, obscured or confused'. In addition to the notion of 'quality of life' central to the hedonistic criterion, the term can also refer to 'a social judgement about a person's *comparative* worth'.[56] Such reasoning ensured that altruistic motivations were deemed to be of considerable importance in the first 'euthanasia' debate. Williams suggested that 'euthanasia' provided a symbiosis of benefit. The man who was prepared to die for the benefit of others had always been regarded as a hero; was it not equally legitimate for a man to take a similar course of action 'when the person to be rescued' was 'himself'?[57]

Attention was also drawn to the mental and physical strain and suffering which the families of the terminally ill were often forced to endure. Those who were in the unfortunate position of having to stand by absolutely helpless while a loved one was tortured to death by a lingering disease.

[W]ho have had to watch, and feebly minister to, throughout long months, a suffering parent, brother, sister, or child; the patient, all this weary while, getting no respite from fierce pain, except in the brief intervals of feverish broken sleep: who have had to witness all this, with the full knowledge that recovery was impossible; with the knowledge, too, that the patient knew his fate as well as the watcher did: knew that there was no hope of relief but in death, and that death was to be reached only by the gradual exhaustion of the bodily strength; with the knowledge, too, that the last living moments would probably be the hardest to bear of all, and might possibly culminate in almost unimaginable horror.[58]

Of course the sense of being a burden upon one's family and friends may augment the patient's suffering and thereby affect his personal quality of life. We must be clear, however, that this is quite distinct from the notions of altruism, obligation and duty which were so evident among the early advocates of 'euthanasia'. Such notions approximate the 'comparative social worth' concept of the 'quality of life' rather than the patient-centred concept of 'quality of life'.

Indeed, it has been suggested that the 'moral response' of most prominent Victorian intellectuals was characterised as much by a culture of 'altruism' as it was by rational calculation of self-interest. '[M]orality was understood very much as a system of obligations ... Victorian moralists exhibited an obsessive antipathy to selfishness, and consequently their reflections were structured by a sharp and sometimes exhaustive polarity between egoism and altruism.'[59] This is a view which receives strong empirical support from a study of the first 'euthanasia' debate.

Yet, for some the idea that 'euthanasia' might be prompted by altruistic considerations has provided considerable cause for concern. Subliminal or overt pressures might act upon a patient to opt for 'euthanasia' when he would not otherwise have done so. If the patient senses that he is a burden to others he may feel *obliged* to end his life. Referring to the case of a patient for whom recovery was an impossibility and for whom suffering was likely to be both severe and protracted, Williams posed the question of whether it was 'not a man's duty to consider others' feelings, and to weigh others' endurance as well as his own; and to bethink himself whether he ought to condemn those nearest to him to witness sufferings which they would find it almost as easy to bear themselves as to see another bear'.[60] 'Euthanasia' was not only a compassionate method of escape for the suffering patient. For the excessively burdensome it had a normative dimension.

The use of the term 'euthanasia' replete with its strong contemporary medical associations appears to have led some commentators to isolate the issue from the broader question of 'justifiable suicide'; a tendency which has produced a number of rather myopic accounts. It seems appropriate therefore to enquire whether the issue of suicide more generally held much currency at this time. Olive Anderson's comprehensive study of *Suicide in Victorian and Edwardian England*[61] suggests that this was indeed the case. 'Among the cultured few, counter-currents flowing from the Enlightenment and Romanticism were making suicides "for love" and those "with a philosophic flavour" acceptable … and for them, the morality of suicide became merely a matter of circumstances.'[62] 'The late Victorian and Edwardian revolt in matters moral and aesthetic thus very definitely included suicide within its scope.'[63]

Lionel Tollemache was particularly keen to draw attention to such shifts. One indication of this was that Archbishop Whately had suggested that suicide was less culpable than the behaviour of the 'prolonged idler'.[64] In taking his own life the suicide deprived society of his services, but the idler was a 'living burden', contributing nothing of value to society while consuming scarce resources.[65] Advancing his own crude utilitarian calculus Tollemache noted that:

> [T]he idle or frivolous man or woman is allowed to spread the infection of idleness and frivolity all around. The drunkard wears out his own constitution, and is of but doubtful profit to his neighbours; yet even he (so long as he only tipples at home) is unrestrained either by the Legislature … Who then has a right to coerce that less objectionable member of society, the would-be suicide? If we may not interfere with the do-nothing-eat-all (or even drink-all), how can we meddle with the do-nothing-eat-nothing?[66]

Having given some indication that there were such things as useless lives, and having intimated that suicide in such cases should not be condemned, Tollemache suggested that 'euthanasia' was a humane method of neutralising the counter-selectivity of medicine which frustrated the efficiency of natural selection. An 'unhealthy, unhappy, and useless man' was effectively 'hustling out' someone who would probably be 'happier, healthier, and more useful than himself'. In making this observation Tollemache was conscious that he might be on dangerous ground. He recognised that similar reasoning might be used to justify the Spartan practice of selective infanticide for weak children. Yet he believed the two cases differed markedly. The 'crushing' objection to infanticide was that the practice was susceptible to abuse. '[A]nti-social consequences might also result. It is possible that, under such a system, full-grown sons might sometimes turn the tables on their aged parents, and inquire concerning them what, not long ago, a young child asked an elderly relative, namely, whether "it would not soon be time for her to go to heaven".'[67]

The 'wild' difference which Tollemache perceived between the two cases was not appreciated by everyone. The article elicited strong concern from the editor of *The Spectator* who suggested that the strongest arguments for extinguishing human suffering were equally applicable to cases of human suffering where there was no possibility of securing the sufferer's consent. These arguments applied to the 'idiotic' and to 'cases of lingering paralysis, where the power of communication between the patient and the outer world is quite cut off, and yet the vegetable functions of the body appear to go on without any hope of the return of the intelligent powers'.[68] Clearly if one was to adopt 'suffering' as the criterion for determining whether life was worthwhile, this could apply to incompetent as well as competent patients. A third party would simply be required to act in the 'best interests' of the patient by securing the minimisation of their suffering by whatever means. This is perhaps the first concrete example of the 'slippery-slope' or 'thin end of the wedge' argument which has appeared with striking regularity throughout the twentieth century.

It was suggested that Mr Tollemache's 'Cure For Incurables' sanctioned 'the right of bystanders to take the destinies of sufferers who have lost all chance of declaring their own wish to themselves, into their hands'.[69] Such an eventuality, it was claimed, would produce a profound shift in the moral attitude of society, the most notable manifestation of which would be 'impatience of hopeless suffering instead of tenderness towards it ... and further, a disposition to regard people as "selfish" who continued burdens upon others without any near and clear chance of the complete restoration of their powers'.[70] Taken to its logical conclusion Tollemache's 'duty' of suicide would apply not only to the sick but to anyone whose existence was the 'cause of more pain than pleasure to others and himself'.[71] In fact similar sentiments had been expressed in *The Saturday Review* the previous year, where it was suggested that there was a difficulty of knowing where to draw the line. If man was subject to the restraint of no moral principle, and was free from consideration of such matters as the 'general sense of security and justice, it can hardly be doubted that a very extensive massacre might be arranged which would be productive of highly beneficial effects to the survivors'.[72]

Having elaborated on what it believed were the 'logical' consequences implicit in Tollemache's article, *The Spectator* conceded that he had not expressly developed these ideas. Indeed in a letter to *The Spectator* Tollemache stated that he had tried to make it absolutely clear that he 'disapproved of such relief ever being given without the dying man's express consent'.[73] It seems that he supported the view that the sufferer should be permitted to shape his own conception of 'worthwhile life', albeit suffused with a sense of duty which suggests that this conception should be determined at least in part by 'comparative social worth'.

Three years after the publication of Tollemache's essay, the ardent birth control campaigner and socialist Annie Besant produced an essay on 'euthanasia'. By this time Besant had come to doubt her Christianity and would later become a prominent figure within the National Secular Society.[74] Her essay on euthanasia was published in a collection of theological pamphlets which seems to have evoked no apparent response. Besant sought to assess the morality of an act in terms of its contribution to society as a whole, claiming that there was a 'wide line of demarcation' between 'euthanasia' and suicide. While both were deaths chosen voluntarily, there was a fundamental difference in the motives prompting the acts. People who commit suicide 'render themselves useless to society for the future' depriving it of their services, and 'selfishly' avoiding the duties 'which ought to fall to their share'. While Besant clearly believed that suicide was justly condemned as a 'crime against society'[75] she believed that the considerations which urged against suicide actually encouraged 'euthanasia'. This was because the sufferor knows that he 'is lost to society', he knows that he is incapable of serving his fellow man in any useful capacity, and moreover recognises that 'he is depriving society of the services of those who uselessly exhaust themselves for him, and is further injuring it by undermining the health of its healthy members'. In such circumstances he is perfectly justified in yielding one last service to society by 'relieving it from a useless burden'. For Besant the individual's life was in a sense the 'property of the state'. In a quasi-Aristotelian argument she suggested that

> The infant is nurtured, the child is educated, the man is protected by others; and, in return for the life thus given, developed, preserved, society has a right to demand from its members a loyal, self-forgetting devotion to the common weal. ... And, when we have given all we can, when strength is sinking, and life is failing, when pain racks our bodies, and the worse agony of seeing our dear ones suffer in our anguish, tortures our enfeebled minds, when the only service we can render man is to relieve him of a useless and injurious burden, then we ask that we may be permitted to die voluntarily and painlessly, and so to crown a noble life with the laurel-wreath of a self-sacrificing death.[76]

However, if the realities of the modern world had exposed the inadequacies of the sanctity of human life as a coherent ethical concept, for many these limitations were preferable to its substitution by a code of ethics based on a crude profit and loss assessment of an individual's contribution to society.

These sentiments were also explored in an article published in *The Contemporary Review* which examined how people 'at different stages of culture' had 'dealt with the aged in their last infirmity'.[77] It noted that the differences between the 'moral rules of higher races' depended 'less on abstract ethical ideas than on the unlike conditions of life among savages and civilised men'.[78] 'In the hand-to-mouth conditions of the rudest savagery', characterised by considerable mobility, it was simply impractical to care for the old people after they had fallen into 'infirmity' and 'imbecility', it was a burden which the community could not bear. South American forest tribes thus regarded the killing of the 'sick and aged a family duty'. Indeed it was not uncommon for them to make full use of the bodies by eating them. According to the article, classical records showed that various barbaric peoples in Asia and Europe kept up the savage practice within historical times. Such were the Massagetae, of whom Herodotus relates, that when a man is extremely old, his assembled relations slay him and boil him with other meat for a feast, holding this the happiest kind of death; or the Sardinians, whose law, according to Aelian, was for the sons to kill with clubs their aged fathers and bury them, considering it shameful to live on in bodily decrepitude.[79]

But when a nation was able to settle into an 'agricultural state' and once it had achieved a modicum of wealth and comfort, the 'excuses' for the 'slaying' of the aged evaporated. Advancing civilisation was characterised by a growing sense that there was a sacredness to life over and above its 'use and pleasure'. After a protracted 'trial', the old 'short' method of dealing with suffering and discomfort was surrendered. It was therefore somewhat peculiar to note that the supporters of euthanasia were seemingly oblivious to the fact that they were proposing to resurrect with 'modern refinements ... the very "cure for incurables" which belonged to ancient savagery, but which has been so consistently rejected by modern civilisation, that not one European in ten knows that it prevailed among his forefathers'.[80] The article suggested that the absence of a 'duty of suicide' in modern society was a laudable indication of man's ethical advance. Ethical progress did not lie in a regression to the practices of savage societies.

Others were evidently of a different mind. Published directly below Tollemache's reply to *The Spectator* was a letter from Francis W. Newman, Emeritus Professor of Latin at University College London,[81] brother of J. H. Newman and a man with distinctive views on a whole host of subjects including the abolition of slavery, temperance, vegetarianism and women's suffrage.[82] Newman had written his letter at the request of Tollemache who believed that he had something of interest to say about the matter. Having endorsed the notion of a 'duty of suicide' Newman's letter went on to advance ideas which were peculiarly similar to those from which Tollemache had attempted to extricate himself. A letter more designed to restore ambiguity to the 'euthanasia' question one would find difficult to conceive. It suggested that, 'If the present discussion should lead to freer avowals, without fear of odium, it will be valuable. I should like to have the Commissioners who visit lunatic asylums called on authoritatively for their sincere opinions of the subject.'[83] Although Newman did not elaborate on this idea, the implication seems to have been that mental defect rendered life less than worthwhile. The origins of Newman's ideas must remain a matter of speculation. One could certainly construct an account which saw his remarks as the product of a considered appraisal of the state of psychiatry in nineteenth-century Britain. We could suggest that he was acutely aware of the apparent failings of the therapeutic asylum, and was perturbed by the seemingly unstoppable rise in the number of asylum inmates. But to suggest that such concerns provided the rationale for Newman's suggestion of extending euthanasia to 'lunatics' would seem rather artificial and excessively deterministic. Newman was not a medical man and he made no allusions to such developments. Concerns of this nature, were however, expressed later on in the century, and will be pursued in the following chapter.

Perhaps Newman's remarks were based upon a profit-and-loss assessment of asylum patients. This suggestion was certainly made in a letter to *The Spectator* which saw Newman's comments as providing confirmation that 'the importance attached to utilitarian consequences as compared with the awe excited by spiritual instincts, is rapidly increasing'.[84] The 'euthanasiasts'' logic seemed to imply that everyone should make an assessment of whether they were a net 'benefit' or 'burden' to society. 'The reaction against the theology which makes obedience and submissiveness the first of virtues, goes much too far when it encourages us to take into our hands the discretion of giving up life itself, – on the strength of a blind and probably worthless calculation of the profit-and-loss account which the remainder of life is likely to yield.'[85] Alternatively, we might argue that Newman's remarks were rooted more philosophically. It is indeed plausible that what was being advocated was a conception of 'worthwhile life' based upon the unimpaired functioning of the brain, upon 'consciousness' or 'rationality'. This is certainly a conception which has found strong expression during the twentieth century with regard to questions of abortion, infanticide and euthanasia, all of which, to some degree, can be seen to depend upon the same underlying ethical issues.

Until now we have made no reference to the practice of 'euthanasia' essentially because this has been a discussion of a debate, but it is also hardly surprising bearing in mind the illegality of euthanasia and the consequent dearth of data. Nevertheless, it is perhaps instructive to note the remarks of a letter to *The Spectator* with regard to a 'widespread' view among many of the 'lower-middle and labouring classes' although seldom 'expressed above a whisper' that patients in hospitals and other institutions who suffered from the advanced stages of syphilis and 'hydrophobic disease' were 'systematically suffocated to get them out of the way'.[86] Whether 'euthanasia' for the diseased in mind was in fact practised we cannot say, nor are we able to say whether it was prompted by a desire to rid society of the burdensome, to reduce unnecessary suffering or because the diseased in mind were considered less than human. It is, however, a theme to which we shall return in the following chapter.

We might also note the remarks of Besant on a matter which was not unrelated. She drew attention to instances of painful disease in which it was quite normal to 'produce partial or total unconsciousness by the injection of morphia, or by the use of some other anaesthetic'. She presented the case of a patient who received this form of treatment, while dying from a tumour in the oesophagus. The patient's sufferings were so pronounced as to bring him close to madness. Consequently, for several weeks prior to his death he was heavily sedated, 'kept in a state of almost complete unconsciousness'. According to Besant, although the patient was breathing he was 'practically dead' for a number of weeks before the candle of existence was finally snuffed. She remarked that '[w]e cannot but wonder, in view of such a case as his, what it is that people mean when they talk of "life"'.[87] For Besant 'life' included

> not only the involuntary animal functions, such as the movements of heart and lungs; but consciousness, thought, feeling, emotion. Of the various constituents of human life, surely those are not the most 'sacred' which we share with the brute, however necessary these may be as the basis on which the rest are built.[88]

The implication was that 'worthwhile life' was not implicit in all 'living' humans, rather it was dependent upon 'rationality', upon that entity constituting a person as opposed to a living organism. This was not notably different from the Lockean notion of a 'person' the attributes of which are 'awareness of one's own existence at different times and places'.[89] This is an important theme which will recur throughout the book.

While Besant's discussion was certainly articulate, her reasoning was perhaps somewhat misplaced in terms of the hypothetical case which she had presented. After all the patient's loss of consciousness was a function of the application of the drug. Her argument of course has much more force in a contemporary setting as a consequence of the development of life-sustaining treatments and technology. It is only in the latter part of the twentieth century that a 're-location' of life from the heart to the brain has been deemed necessary.[90]

This review of the first 'euthanasia' debate has indicated that the concept of 'euthanasia' is not a monolithic one. While Williams, Tollemache and Besant had done much to displace its classical meaning, replacing it with the notion of justifiable mercy-killing, the proposed recipients and the limits of this practice were rather ill-defined. Exactly what life it was justifiable to extinguish was unclear. This ambiguity was in large measure a consequence of the questioning of the Christian doctrine of the sanctity of human life which for many was increasingly seen to be an anachronism in the modern world. Once the concept of the inviolability of human life was brought into question, there emerged a plethora of necessarily subjective conceptions of worthwhile life thereby destroying the basis for consensus. In addition this survey has hopefully gone some way to overturning the temptation to project the late twentieth-century concept of 'euthanasia', which for many is regarded as the tightly defined practice of voluntary physician-assisted suicide, onto what has in fact been a far more complicated debate. In this way it has built upon Van Der Sluis's remark that the 'euthanasia' question has been characterised by a 'powerful undercurrent in favour of the suppression of defective and old people, even against their will'.[91] In so doing the chapter hopes to have highlighted a number of important philosophical themes concerning assessments of the 'worth' of life and the subjective nature of 'euthanasia' which would seem to raise the questions: a 'good death' for whom? and from whose perspective? These themes will be pursued throughout the study.

Notes

1   The titles of these essays were: 'Hold fast your colonies': 'The relation of universities to practical life'; 'Some thoughts on pauperism': 'The natural

history of law; 'The future of women'; 'Euthanasia'; and 'Method and medicine'.

2   *Essays of the Birmingham Speculative Club* (London, 1870).

3   *Ibid.*, preface.

4   Stephan Collini, *Public Moralists: Political Thought and Intellectual Life in Britain 1850–1930* (Oxford, 1991, paperback 1993) p. 53.

5   Christopher Kent, 'Higher journalism and the mid-Victorian clerisy', *Victorian Studies*, 13 (1969) pp. 181–98.

6   *The Saturday Review*, 12 Nov. 1870, pp. 632–4.

7   Collini, *Public Moralists*, p. 53.

8   Circumstantial evidence suggests that Williams was a school teacher, but apart from this there is very little further information about him except that he also published an essay on 'Trade Depression and the Appreciation of Gold' (Birmingham, 1886).

9   S. D. Williams, 'Euthanasia', *Essays by Members of the Birmingham Speculative Club* (London, 1870).

10   Williams, 'Euthanasia', p. 3.

11   Extract from the Western Mail, 28 Feb. 1872 by Mrs Rose Crawshay in her Preface to the fourth edition of 'Euthanasia' by S. D. Williams, reprinted from *Essays by Members of the Birmingham Speculative Club* (London, 1873) p.viii.

12   *Ibid.*

13   See F. H. Sandbach, *The Stoics* (London, 1975, second edn 1989, reprinted 1994) pp. 28–68 and Ranaan Gillon, 'Suicide and voluntary euthanasia: historical perspective', in A. B. Downing (ed.), *Euthanasia and the Right to Die* (London, 1969).

14   W. Bruce Fye, 'Active euthanasia: an historical survey of its conceptual origins and introduction into medical thought', *Bulletin of the History of Medicine*, 1968, pp. 493–502; I. Van Der Sluis, 'The movement for euthanasia 1875–1975', *Janus* Vol. 66, pp. 131–72; Ezekiel J. Emanuel, 'The history of euthanasia debates in the United States and Britain', *Annals of Internal Medicine*, 15 Nov. 1994, Vol. 121, No. 10, pp. 793–802.

15   Williams, 'Euthanasia', p.1.

16   *Ibid.*

17   *Ibid.*, p.2

18   *Ibid.*

19   *Ibid.*

20   Defined in its classical sense.

21   Joseph Bullar, 'On the use of small doses of opium in the act of dying from phthisis', *Assoc. Med. J. London*, 1856, p. 256.

22   *British Medical Journal*, Vol. 2, 7 Jul. 1866, p. 10.

23   *Ibid.*, p. 11.

24   'Euthanasia', *The Spectator*, 18 Mar. 1871, p. 314.

25   *Ibid.*, p. 315.

26   Genesis I: 24–8.

27   Jalland, *Death in the Victorian Family*, p. 21.

28   Owen Chadwick, *The Secularization of the European Mind in the Nineteenth Century* (Cambridge [1975], 1995) p. 37.

29   See Jalland, *Death in the Victorian Family*, pp. 60–1.

30   Williams, 'Euthanasia', pp. 4–5.

31 David Hume, *On Suicide*, published posthumously in 1784 and reprinted from *The Philosophical Works of David Hume* (eds), T. H. Green and T. H. Gosse (London, 1874–75) in Peter Singer (ed.), *Applied Ethics* (Oxford, 1986) pp. 19–27.

32 *Ibid.*

33 Ezekiel J. Emanuel, *The Ends of Human Life: Medical Ethics in a Liberal Polity*, (Cambridge, Mass, 1991) pp. 7–13.

34 Williams, 'Euthanasia', p. 9.

35 See Joseph McCabe, *A Biographical Dictionary of Modern Rationalists* (London, 1920) p. 803.

36 For a brief summary of the relationship between the Athenaeum club and Victorian intellectual life see Collini, *Public Moralists*, pp. 13–21.

37 *Fortnightly Review*, London, Feb. 1873, pp. 218–30. The essay was subsequently published in a collection of essays by Tollemache entitled *Stones of Stumbling* (London, 1884).

38 Kent, 'Higher journalism', p. 192.

39 Tollemache, *Stones of Stumbling*, p. 2.

40 *Ibid.*, p. 5.

41 *Ibid.*, p. 7.

42 For a brief and lucid discussion of the doctrine of double effect, see Helga Kuhse, 'Euthanasia' in Peter Singer (ed.), *A Companion to Ethics* (Oxford, 1995) pp. 300–1.

43 Tollemache, *Stones of Stumbling*, pp. 6–8.

44 *Ibid.*, p. 14.

45 Jose Harris, *Private Lives Public Spirit: Britain 1870–1914* (Oxford [1993], 1994) pp. 150–77.

46 Peter Bowler, *Charles Darwin: The Man and his Influence* (First published 1990 by Blackwell, reissued by Cambridge University Press, 1996) p. 19.

47 Charles Darwin, *Notebooks, 1836–1844*, ed. Paul H. Barrett *et al.*, cited in Peter Singer, *Rethinking Life and Death* (Oxford, 1995) pp. 169–70.

48 Chadwick, *The Secularization of the European Mind*, p. 161.

49 Harris, *Private Lives*, pp. 225–6.

50 Peter J. Bowler, *The Fontana History of the Environmental Sciences* (London, 1992) pp. 308–9.

51 Williams, 'Euthanasia', p. 17.

52 *Ibid.*, p. 20.

53 *Ibid.*, p. 10.

54 *Ibid.*, p. 4.

55 *Ibid.*, pp. 5–6.

56 Emanuel, *The Ends of Human Life*, p. 72.

57 Williams, 'Euthanasia', pp. 7–8.

58 *Ibid.*, p. 3.

59 Collini, *Public Moralists*, pp. 63–5.

60 Williams, 'Euthanasia', p. 10.

61 Olive Anderson, *Suicide in Victorian and Edwardian England* (Oxford, 1987).

62 *Ibid.*, pp. 193–4.

63 *Ibid.*, p. 245.

64 On Whately see, Pietro Corsi, *Science and Religion: Baden Powell and the Anglican Debate, 1800–1860* (Cambridge, 1988).

65 Tollemache, *Stones of Stumbling*, pp. 16–17.

66 *Ibid.*, pp. 17–18.
67 Tollemache, *Stones of Stumbling*, pp. 21–2.
68 'Mr Tollemache on the right to die', *The Spectator*, 15 Feb. 1873, p. 206.
69 *The Spectator*, 15 Feb. 1873, p. 206.
70 *Ibid.*
71 *Ibid.*
72 *The Saturday Review*, 13 Jul 1872, p.43.
73 'Letters to the Editor, The limits of euthanasia', *The Spectator*, 22 Feb. 1873, p. 240.
74 Olivia Bennett, *Annie Besant* (London, 1988).
75 Annie Besant, *Euthanasia* (London, 1875) pp. 18–20.
76 *Ibid.*
77 Edward B. Tylor, 'Primitive society', *The Contemporary Review*, 1873, Vol. 21, pp. 701–18.
78 *Ibid.*, p. 704.
79 *Ibid.*, pp. 704–5.
80 Tylor, 'Primitive society', pp. 704–6.
81 See *Who Was Who*, 1996, A. & C. Black (Publishers) Ltd, CD Rom; *Dictionary of National Biography*, 1995, Oxford University Press, CD Rom.
82 See William Robbins, *The Newman Brothers* (London, 1966) pp. 140–64; Brian Harrison, *Drink and the Victorians* (London, 1971) pp. 159–98; Boyd Hilton, *The Age of Atonement: The Influence of Evangelicalism on Social and Economic Thought, 1785–1865* (Oxford, 1988) pp. 272–81; Colin Spencer, *The Heretic's Feast: A History of Vegetarianism* (London, 1993) pp. 274–7.
83 *The Spectator*, 22 Feb. 1873, p. 240.
84 *Ibid.*, p. 237.
85 *Ibid.*, p. 238.
86 *The Spectator*, 22 Feb. 1873, p. 241.
87 Besant, 'Euthanasia', p.12.
88 *Ibid.*, pp. 12–13.
89 Singer, *Rethinking Life and Death*, p. 180.
90 See: Tomas J. Silber, 'Introduction: bioethics and the paediatrician', *Paediatric Annals*, 10 (1981), 381–2. Cited in Ezekiel J. Emanuel, *The Ends of Human Life*, pp. 10–11.
91 *Van Der Sluis*, 'The movement for euthanasia', p. 168.

2

'Euthanasia' and the medical profession

The 'euthanasia' debate of the 1870s was essentially philosophical. It had taken place in the gentlemanly periodicals of Victorian Britain between a small number of contributors who had no apparent connection with the medical profession. Yet, it was a debate with enormous practical bearing. In pointing out that physicians employed anaesthetics to render their patients unconscious, the interference of medicine with Divine Providence had been laid bare. Attention had also focused on developments in analgesia, which had seemed to blur the distinction between relieving suffering and precipitating death. These observations had driven at the heart of medical ethics, highlighting an apparent contradiction in the Hippocratic Oath; namely its injunction to relieve pain, but not to do the patient any harm. Samuel Williams had taken this a stage further by arguing that in particular circumstances the only way to achieve a 'good death' would be to extinguish a patient's conscious-ness on a permanent basis. Williams's proposal clearly constituted a profound reformulation of the physician's duty, yet historical accounts of the 'euthanasia' movement have done little to elucidate the precise nature of the physician's role vis-à-vis the dying patient. Indeed, they have fundamentally misrepresented the way in which the medical profession perceived the concept of 'euthanasia' in the late nineteenth century.

According to particular commentators, the publication of Williams's essay had succeeded in arousing considerable interest amongst nineteenth-century physicians, prompting 'much discus-sion'.[1] Others have spoken of the regularity with which 'papers, essays, and letters' pertaining to 'euthanasia' appeared in medical as well as non-medical periodicals after 1870.[2] These interpretations find little vindication in the present chapter. In part this confusion has resulted from a failure to provide sufficient demarcation between the nineteenth-century medical discourses of Great Britain and the United States. In America we find that discussion of mercy-killing for the terminally ill took root at a relatively early stage. In Britain, on the other hand, the concept of mercy-killing failed, quite manifestly, to make any impact within the medical profession until shortly before the turn of the twentieth century.

Confusion also seems to have arisen because of the problematic nature of the term 'euthanasia'. Previous commentators have given the impression that after 1870 the term had become synonymous with the notion of physician-assisted suicide. This is of course the notion of 'euthanasia' with which most of us in the late twentieth century are familiar. A patient suffering from an incurable condition solicits the help of a physician to bring his life to a premature conclusion. Discussion of this issue amongst the nineteenth-century medical profession and the broader intellectual population was, however, negligible. If we are to reconstruct matters with any degree of satisfaction we must acknowledge that until at least the turn of the century the term retained a multiplicity of different meanings. Perhaps the most notable of which was the notion of a 'good death'. We can certainly locate medical discussion concerning the mechanisms which the physician might employ to secure a 'good death' for his patient, but this did not include the wilful precipitation of death. Indeed, it will be argued that one of the principal reasons why nineteenth-century physicians were not engaged in discussion about the physician-assisted suicide variety of 'euthanasia' was because they were directing their attention to issues of palliative care which would secure 'euthanasia' in the classical sense.

In fact, it is not until 1901 that we witness the first full-scale advocacy of mercy-killing to emanate from within the British medical profession. To add a further tier of complexity, we should note that the proposals of Dr C. E. Goddard made no use of the term 'euthanasia'.[3] Despite this, it seems clear that his proposal of voluntary mercy-killing, for patients suffering from malignant disease, approximated to modern-day notions of 'euthanasia' far more closely than those instances where the term was used quite explicitly, but where the classical meaning was retained. Perhaps not surprisingly, this pivotal text has been neglected by previous commentators who have allowed their studies to be dictated by an unwavering pursuit of the instances in which the term 'euthanasia' was used. Unfortunately this has produced a number of rather anaemic accounts.

In neglecting this important text these studies have also failed to draw attention to the third form of 'euthanasia' with which this chapter is concerned; the non-voluntary killing of mental defectives. This was a proposal which Goddard placed alongside his suggestions for voluntary mercy-killing. It is also an issue which deserves a far more central place in the history of the 'euthanasia' movement than it has received hitherto. To explain the emergence of such proposals, however, we must set medicine in a broader context, rather than focusing solely upon its efforts to cure the specific ailments of particular individuals. By the late nineteenth century, medicine, health and fitness were associated not only with the individual, but increasingly with society as a whole. We noted in the previous chapter, for example, that the rhetoric of the early supporters of euthanasia was heavily suffused with social Darwinian ideas about the counter-selectivity of modern society. Attention had been drawn to the disadvantageous consequences of the restrictions which civilised society imposed upon the struggle for existence. It had also been made clear, that to remove these restrictions without casting aside altruistic and sympathetic values was impossible. In the present chapter we can trace a radicalisation of these ideas amongst particular individuals. We can identify a heightened readiness to adopt various forms of intervention in order to reverse the counter-selectivity of modern society, thereby curtailing the perceived problem of racial deterioration. Particularly pronounced, were concerns regarding the incidence of mental deficiency, and it is the contention of this chapter that such concerns served to elicit negative eugenic proposals which then fed into proposals for mercy-killing.

This discussion of 'euthanasia' in the late nineteenth and early twentieth centuries is therefore composed of three separate phenomena: the classical notion of a 'good death', physician-assisted suicide, and the non-voluntary killing of mental defectives. Of course these concepts were not always of a mutually exclusive nature. Indeed, there was considerable overlap between them. It is such overlap which has, in no small measure, accounted for the difficulty of mapping the contours of the 'euthanasia' debate during this period. Nevertheless, it is certainly possible to identify a real tradition of discussion about 'euthanasia', albeit in a more complex form than others have acknowledged.

There are several reasons why we might assume medical interest in the dying process to have developed during the course of the late nineteenth and early twentieth centuries. Firstly, there were shifts in mortality patterns which affected the experience of death quite markedly. There was a gradual change from 'infancy to old age as the most probable time of death' which dates 'initially from the late Victorian period.'[4] Broad shifts of this nature had the effect of normalising death, allowing it 'to be perceived as a natural and timely event concluding a long life'.[5] With the aid of developments in disease theory, death was also seen increasingly as the product of a particular disease arising from specific worldly phenomena, rather than as a function of Divine Providence.

It is also reasonably clear that prior to the twentieth century, medicine was able to do little to combat disease. With the exception of smallpox inoculations and vaccinations,[6] medicine seems to have played little role in reducing mortality.[7] Improvements in living standards, improved diet and public health innovations were almost certainly more significant.[8] Indeed, the limited curative capacity of medicine did not go unrecognised amongst nineteenth-century physicians. In his Lumleian Lecture to the Royal College of Physicians of 1862, Dr C. J. B. Williams, FRS, 'reminded his colleagues of the uncertainty of their art, with its continuing failures caused by the intractability of certain disease, and the ultimate inevitability of death. "In the case of cholera, for example; as soon as it is the disease it is death."'[9] In such an environment one can hypothesise that the physician would be required to play a more central role in the dying process. If he could not cure his patients, he could at least make death more comfortable.

Indeed, it has been argued that the approach of nineteenth-century doctors to their dying patients represented a sharp turn away from the 'heroic' attempts to cure the patient, which had allegedly characterised the eighteenth century. Replacing this was a more sympathetic approach with a greater emphasis on palliative care.[10] This alteration in the physician's duty has been termed the doctrine of 'conservatism'. The eighteenth-century methods of sweating, purging and blood-letting were replaced by a philosophy which sought to strike a happier balance between efforts to cure the patient and minimising his suffering. Such a stark transition, however, seems rather caricatured.

The notion of the eighteenth-century physician neglecting issues of palliative care because he was too busy 'physicking people to death' is 'bizarrely implausible'.[11] To suggest that physicians were concerned solely with the prolongation of life regardless of the levels of suffering involved is clearly an exaggeration. We might note that particular physicians such as Dr John Ferriar, Physician to the Manchester infirmary, had stated quite explicitly that 'the physician will not torment his patient with unavailing attempts to stimulate the dissolving system, from the idle vanity of prolonging the flutter of the pulse for a few mere vibrations'.[12] He stated that 'When all hopes of revival are lost, it is still the duty of the physician to soothe the last moments of his existence.' The physician should be at liberty to 'determine when officiousness becomes torture'. We should also be aware that the eighteenth century had witnessed a considerable increase in the consumption of strong narcotic substances. The use of opium, laudanum and alcohol all rose quite markedly, which undoubtedly served to ease many deaths. Nevertheless, it seems likely that subscription to a 'doctrine of conservatism', which required the physician to devote more attention to issues of palliative care, was more a characteristic of nineteenth-century medicine than it was of the eighteenth century. A 'utilitarian approach to ethics and its statistical effort to quantify a precise balance between helping and avoiding harm distinguished conservative professionalism from its predecessors'.[13]

The physician's heightened concern with the deathbed experience of his patient was, according to Bruce Fye, underlined by significant advances which were made in diagnosis, prognosis and pathology. Making reference to medical innovations such as Pierre Louis's introduction of statistical methods and the 'emphasis on pathological correlations of clinical conditions', Fye has argued that the physician was provided with the mechanisms to 'prognosticate more accurately than ever before'. Although prognosis was certainly not precise, 'there was a growing body of scientifically derived information upon which a physician could rely in making diagnostic and prognostic decisions'. Fye claims that, 'Only when a patient's condition could be judged incurable with reasonable accuracy would it be feasible to propose a concept as radical as "active" euthanasia.'[14] Discussion of this nature is certainly not redundant as a method of contextualisation, but although the notion of a 'doctrine of conservatism' seems tenable, discussion of 'active euthanasia' was by no means a logical by-product.

In this respect we might return to the remarks of Dr C. J. B. Williams, who despite conceding medicine's limited curative potential also recognised that significant improvements had been made in methods of care for terminally ill patients; ensuring that the physician's role in the dying process was regarded highly. 'I speak of the Prolongation and Utilization of Life, and the Alleviation of Suffering. These may seem very subordinate at first, but often they are far from being so in the estimation of the patient.'[15] In fact, it would seem that throughout the nineteenth century there were several prominent physicians expert in palliative care, none of whom was prepared to advocate the wilful destruction of incurable patients.

Perhaps the most notable of these was the Royal Physician, Sir Henry Halford, who was alleged to be 'so suave' in 'his bedside manner that aristocratic women were said to prefer dying with Sir Henry than living with lesser physicians'.[16] Halford provides the classic example of a physician who made use of an array of soporific drugs in order to secure a peaceful and painless death for his patients, becoming 'the most sought-after physician of his age precisely because his patients had confidence that through generous medication he would not let them die in agony'.[17] He was also scrupulous in devoting care and attention to his patients' psychological well-being. Where it had been commonplace for the physician to inform the patient of his likely fate, so that he could prepare himself spiritually for death, Halford preferred to retain an air of optimism until the bleak truth could no longer be withheld. Truth was divulged in accordance with the physician's perception of its therapeutic value.[18]

While it seems clear that palliative care was not the subject of total neglect amongst physicians, it was an issue which had tended to be rather eclipsed by other areas of medicine. *The Lancet* certainly lent credence to this view when it noted that in recent times there had been a disproportionate inclination to advance 'the study of pathogeny and that of intimate pathology, while the whole subject of therapeutics, the *ars medendi*, has been too much driven into the background'. This was said to be a rather 'sad reflection'. The article called upon medical practitioners to recall that their place in the social system was 'conceded to them in virtue of their office as healers of the sick and ministers at the bedside. Every other study and medical accomplishment is for them subservient.'[19] This adroit observation was advanced in the review of a 'treatise' by William Munk, fellow and late censor of the Royal College of Physicians. Indeed, if we are to talk about what 'euthanasia' meant to the physician of the nineteenth century it is essential to draw attention to this highly respected 'little book' which was deemed 'not to have a fault'.[20] Peculiarly, Munk's book of 1887, entitled *Euthanasia: or Medical Treatment in Aid of an Easy Death*, has received little attention in the historical accounts of 'euthanasia' despite the fact that it is the only medical work to use that term in its title.

Munk believed that the role of medicine in the dying process needed to be improved. He noted that medical texts tended to neglect discussion of the management of the dying and the most appropriate methods of treatment for the relief of final sufferings. He also lamented the fact that the subject was overlooked in the medical schools. The young physician upon entering his duties was forced to learn for himself what it was best to do, or best not to do. All this 'in the most solemn and delicate position in which he can be placed, in attendance on the dying'.[21] Munk was also keen to point out that death was usually a painless experience, citing such figures as Benjamin Brodie to this effect.[22] While death might be accompanied by a degree of suffering, this was not 'naturally or necessarily incident to the act of dying' rather it was a function of the 'surrounding circumstances that admit of alteration or removal'.[23]

Thus, he drew attention to such matters of importance as the weight of bedclothes in minimising the patient's 'restlessness' and 'jacitation'. Problems were often alleviated by lightening the patient's bedding. Difficulties associated with breathing were frequently remedied by admitting cool, fresh air into the bedchamber and by changing the patient's posture with the aid of pillows to ensure the 'efficient support of the trunk of the body'.[24] The correct administration of nutriment was also deemed to be of considerable importance. Errors in feeding were frequently the cause of much discomfort. The 'sinking and exhaustion that are in progress throughout the system' were commonly followed by the over zealous 'administration of food and stimulants' by well-meaning but misguided attendants. The stomach which shares in the overall exhaustion of the body is unable to cope with such ingestion:

The dying person is induced by the wearisome importunity of his attendants to take food or stimulants, against which nature and his stomach revolt. The evident dislike and loathing with which he submits, the difficulty he has in swallowing it, and urging and retching which that act sometimes induces, ought to save him from what is really under the circumstances an act of cruelty.[25]

The administration of alcohol in its fermented or distilled forms was believed to be a far more sympathetic and effective treatment. Its high 'diffusive power' ensured that it passed rapidly into the blood, stimulating the tiring heart and promoting circulation through the lungs, 'one of its most valuable properties in the dying'. In addition, there was some speculation that the intake of alcohol might aid the secretion of gastric juice and stimulate the peristaltic movements of the stomach, thereby helping the digestive process, supporting 'the patient in the best and most natural manner'.[26] Ice cubes, lemonade and weak black tea with a slice of lemon were similarly recommended in order to combat the inextinguishable thirst often present amongst the dying. Echoing the views of such eminent authorities as the Prussian Professor C. W. Hufeland, Munk noted the importance of opium and laudanum. It is imperative, however, to note his conditions for their application.

Opium is administered to the dying, as an anodyne to relieve pain; or as a cardiac and cordial to allay that sinking and anguish about the stomach and heart, which is so frequent in the dying, and is often worse to bear than pain, however severe. Opium should rarely be administered to the dying as mere hypnotic, or with a view to enforce sleep. *To do so would be to risk throwing the patient into a sleep from which he may not wake.*[27]

Munk leaves us in no doubt that while opium might be used to ease the patient's dying moments, the precipitation of death was unacceptable. It should be administered in its liquid forms, but only when the air passages were free from secreted obstructions: 'so long as there is neither lividity nor even duskiness of face, opium, if indicated, may be given in aid of the Euthanasia; but if they are present, it is hazardous and might hasten death'.[28]

Munk had stated quite eloquently that the 'whole subject of Euthanasia, or of a calm and easy death, in so far as it respects the physician' was 'in need of special study; and of a systematic treatment that has not hitherto been accorded to it'.[29] Yet, one would find it difficult to draw a clearer distinction between the notions of 'euthanasia' as espoused by Samuel Williams and William Munk. While it seems reasonably clear that the medical press was not peppered with articles pertaining to 'euthanasia' of any variety, those which did appear, tended to relate to the classical notion of a 'good death.'

It is not until 1896 that we witness discussion of the mercy-killing variety of 'euthanasia' in the British medical press. In fact two articles discussed the matter that year,[30] but both were concerned with a debate which had taken place in an American context. The Practitioner included an article which alluded to a medico-legal congress held in New York at which a lawyer had claimed that medical practitioners frequently gave incurably diseased patients an overdose of opiates in order to end the agony of their sufferings. The American medical press had apparently denied these claims 'indignantly', noting that conscience and legal sanction ruled out such a practice. Moreover, it was made abundantly clear that the rule of the profession was that laid down in the Hippocratic Oath: 'I will give no deadly medicine to anyone if asked, nor suggest any such counsel.' The doctor's remit was to discover methods of prolonging life, not shortening it.

Although it was conceded that self-destruction in cases of 'hopeless' and 'painful' disease should have no 'legal stigma' attached to it, the ethical principles of the medical profession were clearly voiced. Such practices were diametrically opposed to the 'instincts and traditions' of the physician's art. To grant a medical man the authority to end the lives of suffering patients beyond 'all hope of cure' would be of questionable 'benefit to the community' and would serve to discredit the profession. The article had also drawn a distinction between positive efforts to bring about a patient's death and refraining from the prolongation of life when this could 'only mean protracted agony', however, this is a view which is certainly compatible with the traditional notion of 'euthanasia'. The same distinction is still made by the twentieth-century hospice movement which is of course steadfastly opposed to the concept of physician-assisted suicide.

The British Medical Journal (BMJ) of the following year also drew attention to this issue. It remarked that in the 'last hours' the physician sometimes ceased to 'trouble the sufferer' and in so doing conspired to 'let drop a few hours of life'. The frequency with which such cases presented themselves was, however, fewer than might be supposed. Echoing the comments of Joseph Bullar, it was noted that there was often a form of symbiosis between remedies for relieving pain and prolonging life. 'For instance, the dextrous insertion of a cordial enema may not only prolong life for a few hours, but will also relieve the agony of death.' These were considered to be rather peripheral matters. As the *BMJ* observed, the law 'is not curious to consider the final scene too nearly'. The substantive issue revolved around 'the deliberate cutting of the thread of a life which, if skilfully and assiduously guarded, would last some substantial time', and it was made abundantly clear that such a practice 'would never be accepted by the medical profession'.[31]

Particular historians have suggested that the reason why mercy-killing failed to engage nineteenth-century British physicians, was because they lacked the life-prolonging technology which has made 'euthanasia' an issue of such practical importance in the late twentieth century.[32] This explanation seems less convincing than the simple observation of medical conservatism. Indeed, the air of conservatism which continued to pervade the approach of the physician with regard to the use of narcotic substances at the deathbed scene is quite striking. Pronounced hesitancy still surrounded the ethics of securing 'euthanasia' in the classical sense. A letter sent to *The Lancet* in 1899 by a physician is particularly instructive in this regard:

> Sirs, – Within a few weeks I have had under my care a case of carcinoma uteri extending to the bladder and adjacent parts. The pain accompanying the disease in its later stages was severe and only controlled by strong suppositories of morphia, and the patient's death struggle was an awful and most pitiable experience, lasting certainly three or four days. I tried liquor opii sedatives 10 minims every two hours, but only two or three doses could be swallowed. I seek in this letter information from my *confreres* on the treatment one should adopt in such cases – e.g., would it be justifiable to use morphia hypodermically? or to what extent would the inhalation of chloroform be admissible in mitigation of so great agony and distress?
>
> I am, Sirs, yours faithfully,
> EUTHANASIA.[33]

The anxiety about how far one was justified 'in pushing anodynes and anaesthetics' in such circumstances was acknowledged by *The Lancet* in its reply to the above enquiry. It stated, however, that the physician would have been justified in administering morphia hypodermically. It was also considered legitimate to keep patients under the influence of chloroform in order to mitigate the sufferings which accompanied convulsions. The possibility of giving an overdose to patients who were incurably ill and close to death was also raised. 'No one can deny "that it would be the kindest thing to do".' But is was stated very clearly, that the duty of the physician was 'to attempt to save life, never to destroy it'.[34] If there was reluctance with regard to the employment of particular substances which would relieve the final sufferings, but which could plausibly shorten life by a few hours, the notion of actively and intentionally bringing about a patient's death was absolutely beyond the bounds of acceptable, ethical behaviour.

In 1901, however, a particularly interesting speech was delivered by the Medical Officer of Health for Willesden, Dr C. E. Goddard,[35] before the Willesden and District Medical Society entitled 'Suggestions in Favour of Terminating Absolutely Hopeless Cases of Injury or Disease'.[36] Goddard drew attention to two distinct categories of sufferer for whom he considered mercy-killing desirable. Firstly, there was *Class A* which included the 'hopelessly diseased' who were very likely to die in the near future, although perhaps with an interval of many months of horrendous suffering. These patients would be entitled to 'solicit' the help of a 'Central Committee' to bring their suffering to a swift conclusion. This was the voluntary category, 'they actually demand the relief for themselves'.[37] Attention was drawn to the plight of 'those poor creatures with inaccessible and therefore inoperable malignancy'. It was said that these patients often longed for death and it was common for them to beg their physician not to prolong their torturous existence. This was the first suggestion of its nature to emerge from within the medical profession. If we wish to identify medical phenomena which may have prompted such a proposal at this time, we might note that the number of deaths from cancer had increased quite markedly over the course of the second half of the nineteenth century. In 1847 there were 274 recorded deaths from cancer per million and by 1900 this had reached 800.[38] Whereas infectious diseases tended to carry people off with some rapidity, death from malignant disease tended to be a more protracted experience, thereby lending weight to the argument for a premature conclusion of suffering.

Goddard suggested that when death finally came to the salvation of such pitiable creatures, the friends and family of the patient, regardless of wealth, made use of one phrase '"What a happy release!" and we know that they in saying this are not always disinterested, for they have generally suffered much themselves'.[39] Even in this example of what is commonly known as voluntary euthanasia we find that the benefits to be derived from the application of euthanasia do not pertain solely to the patient, the sufferings of the family and friends were also seen to be important factors by Goddard.

Significantly, Goddard juxtaposed these proposals with proposals for non-voluntary mercy-killing, and it is here that the real novelty of his proposals lay. To some extent we can see his proposals as a development of the social Darwinian remarks which had pervaded the essays of Williams and Tollemache concerning the counter-selectivity of modern society. Indeed, by the 1880s, degeneration as well as progression was seen increasingly as an evolutionary possibility.[40] This was particularly so with regard to the problem of mental defectives, who formed the core of Goddard's *Class B*. Mental defect was a sphere in which in contrast to most areas pertaining to health and fitness,[41] subscription to strict hereditarian views tended to predominate. There was a widespread belief that mental defect was not only incurable, but it got worse over succeeding generations. In the late nineteenth century, concerns about the incidence of mental deficiency had become particularly pronounced, spreading beyond the confines of the medical profession becoming associated increasingly with broader concerns about racial degeneration.

Darwin, for example, had noted that civilised man did 'his utmost to check the process of elimination', building 'asylums for the imbecile, the maimed, and the sick' medicine preserved the weakest and allowed them to reproduce. 'It is surprising how soon a want of care, or care wrongly directed, leads to the degeneration of a domestic race.'[42] He was, however, decidedly reticent about the desirability of intervention to reverse modern society's counter-selectivity. Such action was considered impossible unless one was prepared to reject altruistic and sympathetic values which were themselves the product of the evolution of ethical values.[43] Francis Newman had come perhaps closest to advocating an interventionist approach, when he remarked that he would like to have the opinion of the Lunacy Commissioners regarding the desirability of extending 'euthanasia' to asylum patients. It was the acceptance of the need for various forms of intervention which most clearly set apart the eugenic ideas of the late nineteenth century from the social Darwinian thought which had preceded it, and upon which it was predicated in no small degree. Goddard's proposals for the non-voluntary killing of mental defectives were underpinned to a considerable extent by such eugenic ideas.

When we refer to the field of eugenics, we refer of course to an extremely broad church. The term was coined by Francis Galton,[44] a first cousin of Charles Darwin, who defined it as 'the science which deals with all influences that improve the inborn qualities of the race; also with those that develop them to the utmost advantage'.[45] While it seems rather tangential to explore its many facets, it is necessary to make a few brief, elementary points. At its most basic, eugenic thought stressed the centrality of heredity in determining a man's natural abilities. The offspring of eminent parents were the recipients of their superior qualities, most notably intellectual ability. The offspring of *inferior* stock were similarly furnished with their parents inherent qualities, or lack thereof, which tended to consign them to a much lowlier station in life. Galton had suggested that the procreation of the 'undesirable' was outstripping that of the naturally able with consequent deterioration in the aggregate quality of the human population of Great Britain.

Eugenic prescriptions can be divided into two strands; positive and negative eugenics. Galton and most early eugenists were concerned primarily with the former. They aimed to encourage marriage and greater fertility among the gifted minority. In this chapter, however, we are concerned with negative eugenics, which sought to prevent racial degeneration by restricting the reproduction of the 'unfit'. The 'unfit' was in itself an extremely broad category. The eugenists identified two distinct strata at the lowest end of society.[46] 'One was unambiguously degenerate because of identifiable hereditary abnormalities' the other 'was less obviously dysgenic, but was still undesirable (casual labourers, the unskilled working class, slum-dwellers)'. It should be made clear that this chapter is concerned only with the former category; that is with tangibly defective individuals. This was the group which was 'clustered at the extreme left of the distribution curve, and whose powers of reason and memory were even below those of dogs and other intelligent animals'.[47]

Advocates of negative eugenics tended to concern themselves with reducing fertility among the hereditarily unfit. John Berry Haycraft, professor of physiology at University College Cardiff was one of the first writers to advance ideas urging the adoption of negative eugenic policies in Great Britain. Haycraft's *Darwinism and Race Progress,*[48] was concerned with the 'necessity for replacing one selective agency by another'.[49] It was noted that 'microbes' and 'other selective agencies' had once served to sort the wheat from the chaff, securing the improvement of the race. But such continued improvement was no surety. Improvements in scientific method had revealed the possibility of exterminating the microbe, and if the 'selecting microbe' was to disappear, man would have to replace it with the selective method of his 'forethought'. Unless an enlightened mechanism of selection was substituted in place of the microbe 'racial decay' was considered inevitable. Employing Darwinian rhetoric, Haycraft argued that the only sensible option open to man was to apply the same care and attention to his own 'race propagation that a gardener' did 'to his roses or chrysanthemums, or a dog-fancier to his hounds or terriers'.[50] The hereditary 'defective' should be precluded from reproduction by means of segregation.

These concerns were echoed in a book entitled *The Problems of a Great City* by Arnold White published in 1887.[51] Although White was famed for having coined the phrase 'sterilisation of the unfit', he actually stopped short of advocating such a measure because it was impractical and rather severe. In fact he favoured a policy of segregating particular defectives. Like Darwin, Williams, Tollemache and Haycraft, White noted that medical science, 'sanitary precautions, poor laws, vaccination, hospitals, [and] charity' served to mitigate suffering, but thereby preserved the diseased. The destiny of England was seen to depend on 'a struggle between moral and mental enlightenment and mental and physical deterioration'. If it was 'monstrous that the weak should be destroyed by the strong', it was more 'repugnant' to 'instinct and to reason that the strong and capable should be overwhelmed by the feeble, ailing, and unfit'.[52]

Taken to the extreme, eugenic concerns could elicit more draconian measures, the epitome of which we might wish to term 'eugenic euthanasia'. It has been suggested that the concepts of 'euthanasia' and 'eugenics' have a history of strong overlap. Martin Pernick's study of *Eugenics and the Death of Defective Babies*, has made the etymological observation that both terms share the Greek prefix 'eu' meaning 'good'. This he claims provides an indication that both terms are 'deeply value-laden'. More explicitly, both concepts offered assessments of which lives were unworthy of life. '"Eugenics" could mean judging who was "better-not-born", and "euthanasia" could mean deciding who was "better-off-dead".'[53] Thus, while eugenists generally believed that it was more desirable and effective to work through a regulation of the birth rate, eugenic policies could be designed to reduce the number of defectives in society by putting them to death. A measure as extreme as this was highly contentious and understandably eugenic literature in which proposals of this nature were advanced is not plentiful.

The only proposal of a similar nature prior to Goddard's paper of 1901 appears to be that of Oxford metaphysician F. H. Bradley in an article published in the *International Journal of Ethics* in 1894.[54] This was ostensibly concerned with the subject of capital punishment for criminals, but its scope was much broader. Although Bradley did not explicitly advocate the killing of defectives, his comments certainly bowed in that direction. His article is also significant in demonstrating that eugenic ideas were not the preserve of the medical profession. He claimed that particular points of the prevailing moral code were deemed in need of correction, and a reversion to a non-Christian and perhaps 'Hellenic' ideal was mooted. For Bradley, Darwinism dictated a policy of social surgery. Society was an organism from which the diseased parts should be removed, in the same way that the surgeon cuts out cancerous growths from the human body. Individuals were deemed to be of unequal worth, their value was relative. The community constituted its 'own Providence' and therefore the rights of the individual by comparison could not be deemed sacred. Individuals were dispensable if the best interest of the collective dictated such a course of action. Not only was Bradley 'oppressed by the ineffectual cruelty of our imprisonments', he was also

> disgusted at the inviolable sanctity of the noxious lunatic. The right of the individual to spawn without restriction his diseased offspring on the community, the duty of the state to rear wholesale and without limit and unselected progeny - such duties and rights are to my mind a sheer outrage on Providence. A society that can endure such things will merit the degeneracy which it courts.[55]

It was not until Goddard's paper of 1901, however, that anyone really grasped the nettle and fused the concepts of eugenics and euthanasia. It is perhaps instructive to note that Charles Goddard was a future member of the Eugenics Education Society,[56] and would also serve on the Consultative Medical Council of the Voluntary Euthanasia (Legalisation) Society.[57] We should be clear, however, that Goddard was not advocating anything like the wholesale killing of defectives, he was concerned only with the worst cases. These were the individuals that formed the basis of his *Class B*. It would include a substantial number of cases resident in institutions and asylums: 'for example, idiots, beings having only semblance to human form, incapable of improvement and education, unable to feed themselves, or of perceiving when the natural functions are performed, unable to enjoy life or of serving any useful purpose in nature'.[58]

Goddard believed that the arguments for 'nurturing' and caring for 'such creatures' were both inadequate and misguided. Regardless of the cause of the specific defect, whether it was the consequence of an accident, or the product of disease in a 'previous generation' these sufferers were, in Goddard's eyes, 'an insult to God's beautiful creation, and their existence surely should not be tolerated in this, a more enlightened time!'[59] He believed his proposals would at first incorporate only a limited number of persons from *Class B* until a failproof system of classification could be determined. This issue provided the 'chief difficulty', but he was sure that the problem would be soluble in time. After all 'a visit to an Asylum would soon put you in the possession of the facts that would help one to fix limits as to mental calibre and the patients' capability or possibility of improvement; such cases as terminal GPI's (General Paralysis of the Insane) for example, hopeless maniacs, and melancholics, monstrosities, and scores of others.'[60]

Goddard's perception of the asylum as a receptacle for incurable defectives was not unique. In the first half of the nineteenth century there had been an air of optimism about the curative potential of psychiatry. The asylum combined with new philosophical and therapeutic approaches had been seen as a panacea for mental illness. But such enthusiasm began to wane. Eminent figures within the field of psychiatry tended to see the therapeutic function of the asylum giving way to a policy of containment. Such sentiments were evident in a number of Presidential Addresses of the Medico-Psychological Society. Pathological investigations had also failed to reveal the anticipated structural lesions causing mental illness and considerable doubt also hovered over chemotherapeutic methods of treating mental illness. Henry Tuke, the President of 1881 acknowledged that 'Psychological medicine can boast, as yet, of no specifics, nor is it likely, perhaps, that such a boast will ever be made.'[61]

The apparent futility of nineteenth-century psychiatry, was compounded by the overwhelming pressure of numbers which asylums faced. Several presidents of the Medico-Psychological Association[62] were of the opinion that this rise was not the product of an increase in the incidence of insanity, rather it was a function of the redistribution of the mentally ill, combined with population increases and an excess of asylum admissions over deaths. Families who were previously prepared to look after their mentally ill or impaired children and elderly relatives suffering from dementia, now felt the pressures of urban industrial society which tended to make them more ready to seek 'outside care'.

A law of 1874 also provided for the removal of sufferers who had formerly been housed in non-specialist institutions like prisons and workhouses to the asylums. Particular contemporaries were certainly convinced that mental illness was on the increase. Regardless of the causes, there was a clear and incontrovertible rise in the asylum population. In 1847 the number of 'lunatics', 'idiots', and 'persons of unsound mind' in county asylums numbered approximately 5,500,[63] by 1869 this figure had risen to 26,867.[64] As early as '1876, the Lunacy Commissioners – so staunch in their earlier advocacy of the therapeutic benefits of non-restraint – were suggesting that only some seven per cent of the mad were actually, after all, curable'.[65]

Goddard was quite explicit in linking the necessity of his proposed policy of non-voluntary mercy-killing for mental defectives, with the incurability and unrestrained fertility of the unfit.

> I do not see ... much force in the argument that the movement is a retrograde one so long as the need is likely to continue ... Whilst the inter-marriage of the unfit, whether they be alcoholic, syphilitic, phthisical, the morbid in mind and the diseased in body, is permitted – as long as the human race indeed is liable to sin and to accident in all forms, so long I presume there will be but little prospect of diminution, much less of the elimination of these sad terminations.[66]

It is not clear at this point whether Goddard's proposal was entirely isolated, or whether it was in any way typical of negative eugenics. Robert Rentoul's comprehensive eugenic text entitled *Race Culture or Race Suicide? A Plea for the Unborn*[67] is worth mentioning in this regard. Rentoul, a Liverpool physician was perhaps the most outspoken and extreme of the early eugenists. He was renowned for advancing his views with 'a violence of language and a disregard of all the difficulties, which cannot have done his cause any good'.[68] He has also been identified by Pernick as an advocate of infanticide based upon eugenic criteria.

Like many other eugenic texts, Rentoul drew attention to the 'large and increasing number of the insane' in Great Britain. He was certainly well informed, having laid evidence before the Royal Commission on the Care and Control of the Feeble-minded. 'Idiots, imbeciles, feeble-minded, habitual inebriates, lunatics, and habitual criminals' were all deemed to be incurable; they would never be able to produce healthy offspring. Reference was made to the fifty-sixth Annual Report of the Lunacy Commission, which suggested that over the past thirty years, the recovery rate for mental illness had seen no marked improvement. Rentoul believed that the Lunacy Commissioners had failed 'absolutely' because they contented themselves with 'caring for the insane' rather than seeking to 'prevent insanity and mental degeneracy'.[69] Indeed, he was of the opinion that 'lunatics' and 'other degenerates' were effectively encouraged to marry. He believed that man was currently engaged in the manufacture of 'diseased infants, idiots, imbeciles, and the insane'. A 'cowardly policy of *laissez-faire*' had been adopted and shown to be a manifestly inadequate method of preventing an increase in the 'sum total of physical deterioration and mental degeneration'.[70] Even if society were to adopt a policy of raising the minimum age of marriage, and to require a 'pre-nuptial certificate of good health', to make illegal the marriage of degenerates, and to institute a policy of non-intervention with regard to attempted suicides, alongside policies of infanticide, abortion and contraception, there would still remain, 'at the very least, 60,721 publicly recognized idiots, imbeciles, and feeble-minded, 117,272 lunatics, 23,244 criminals, 9,822 deaf and dumb from childhood, 60,000 prostitutes, 62,187 epileptics, 88,347 backward children, and about 18,242 habitual vagrants, all engaged in breeding degenerates'. The 'legacy of degeneracy' was considered to be 'too vast' and 'too deep to be cured by mere palliatives'.[71]

Of all the depressing sights seen by the physician none is so intensely humiliating to our civilization and Christianity than is the Asylum for Idiots and Imbeciles. They are to be pitied, and it is somewhat of a consolation that the onlooker suffers more than do these poor wrecks and products of our blatant and boasting civilization. They make one feel that it is a pity that, when the higher apes 'crossed the rubicon,' so as to become men and women, 'they burned their boats,' and so prevented our degenerate samples of mankind from reverting to the monkey stage of evolution. Such atavism would, however, be hard upon the apes, and it is better that we have to take care of these products of our own misdeeds.[72]

Despite Rentoul's sharp language, Pernick's claim that he favoured a policy of selective infanticide is false. His preferred method for the eradication of degeneracy was eugenic sterilisation. He suggested that if all diseased humanity 'were afflicted with sterility, the present sad conditions would disappear'.[73] According to Rentoul economic considerations alone deemed such a measure desirable. He claimed that national expenditure on the upkeep of degenerates was in the region of thirteen million pounds per annum.[74] But he believed the mercy-killing of such degenerates to be out of the question. His prescription was clear: '"keep everything alive." The murder of degenerates either when inside or outside the uterus is a dangerous and repulsive proposal. Every human being has the inalienable right to live. ... The step from killing the child in the womb to murdering a person outside the womb is a dangerously narrow one.'[75]

Indeed, it appears that Goddard was the only advocate of eugenic killing outside the womb. We should note, however, that Goddard's proposal for the mercy-killing of the mentally ill, and those with mental defects was predicated not only on eugenic grounds, but also – at least to some extent – on humanitarian grounds. As we indicated in Chapter 1, arguments concerning the relief of suffering which are employed to support voluntary euthanasia for the *compos mentis* might also be transferred to the case of mercy-killing for the incompetent. It could be argued that individuals whose lives are racked by pain and suffering should not be denied ultimate relief simply because they are incapable of articulating the desire to die.

Indeed, this is suggested implicitly when we consider precisely which individuals were included in Goddard's *Class B*. They were certainly not mild cases, they included those with no 'will power nor intelligence of their own', who were a 'burden to themselves', friends, and to 'society generally, beings of course absolutely incapable of improvement'.[76] Such individuals would be appraised by a committee of experts and if they were deemed eligible for relief, arrangements would be made for the termination of their 'miserable existence'. This category relates to what we might call non-voluntary euthanasia. As the patient/sufferer is seemingly incapable of making the decision whether or not to curtail their existence by means of euthanasia, a third party is required to do so. Of course one assumes that the third party would attempt to act in the best interests of the patient, for example when extreme suffering is evident, but nevertheless it seems clear that in the case of non-voluntary euthanasia some form of subjective criteria of the worth or value of life must be employed in making this decision. In the categories cited by Goddard it is not at all evident that continual pain and suffering is the key criterion. Indeed it appears that there is a distinct unwillingness to accept as valuable, life which diverges from a narrowly defined subjective ideal.

In employing eugenic concepts, Goddard's paper had suggested that not all life was worthwhile. Life could become of negative value for its bearer and in particular instances there was life which was considered to be frankly undesirable, worthless and dispensable. Such views were extreme and found no support in a medical profession characterised by some degree of conservatism as Britain's was at the turn of the century. Consequently, Goddard's paper appears to have been ignored.

The following year (1902) the term 'euthanasia' was used in its modern sense in a medical text,[77] and the practice was again considered unethical. In 1905, in the course of his farewell speech at Johns Hopkins University before taking up the Regius Chair in Medicine at Oxford, William Osler made reference to Anthony Trollope's novel, *The Fixed Period*, in which all those over sixty would be put to death by chloroform. This produced something of an outcry in the American press,[78] and Osler was forced to make clear that he was not actually advocating such a measure. He had intended this as a humorous remark to go alongside his suggestion that by the age of sixty the majority of professional men had completed their most productive work in life. Osler believed, that 'incalculable benefit', in 'commercial, political' and 'professional' terms would accrue if, 'as a matter of course, men stopped work at this age'.[79] The speech produced little discussion in Britain. The *BMJ* merely commented upon the embarrassing inability of the Americans to take a joke; that such a distinguished professor of medicine would really have proposed a policy of this sort was preposterous.

Indeed it was not until 1906 with a short article in the *BMJ* that the question of euthanasia appears to have stirred people's imaginations. The catalyst for the renewed interest was a Bill which had been submitted to the Iowa State Legislature by a Dr R. H. Gregory. Once again we see proposals for voluntary euthanasia for the terminally ill alongside eugenic concerns. The Bill proposed that 'persons suffering from hopeless disease or injury and hideously deformed or idiotic children should be put out of existence by the administration of an anaesthetic'.[80] The *BMJ* left its readers in no doubt that such proposals were unacceptable: 'That the man is either a crank of a particularly noxious type or a mere notoriety hunter, is clear enough from the statement attributed to him that he simply wishes to make lawful that which is already practised by the greatest physicians and surgeons in every large hospital in the United States.'[81] In addition to the unacceptability of what might be termed 'eugenic euthanasia' strong reservations were advanced with regard to the voluntary practice. Significantly in the light of arguments advanced by Fye, we might note that the *BMJ* was less confident about the infallibility of diagnostic techniques, remarking that 'until science can pronounce a sufferer's doom with absolute certainty, "euthanasia" must always involve a serious risk of murder'.[82] The *BMJ* also noted that the proposal for

> ending by what is euphemistically called euthanasia, sufferings which cannot be mended, is by no means novel. Every now and again it is put forward either by literary dilettanti who discuss it as an academic subtlety, or by neurotic 'intellectuals' whose high-strung temperament cannot bear the thought of pain. The medical profession has always sternly set its face against a measure that would inevitably pave the way to the grossest abuse and would degrade them to the position of executioners.[83]

Excepting this juxtaposition of voluntary euthanasia and non-voluntary euthanasia for defectives in an American context we find no discussion of eugenic euthanasia of the sort advocated by Goddard. Of course it was not until 1907 that eugenic thought acquired an organised forum in Britain with the establishment of the Eugenics Education Society, and when this organisation did appear it was decidedly cautious in its proposals. The idea of mercy-killing as a tool of negative eugenics was probably the most radical measure conceivable and consequently found little outlet within the eugenics movement. Indeed, we might note that even discussion of sterilising the 'unfit' failed to be discussed within the pages of the *BMJ* with any seriousness before 1909; it was seen to be an extreme measure which was likely to offend public opinion and ultimately damage the eugenic cause. From time to time, however, particular figures did embarrass the Society with extreme proposals that served only to taint the image of an organisation about which many people already harboured pronounced suspicion.

In November 1909, for example, the Mayor of Plymouth proposed that the incurably 'feeble-minded' and 'hopelessly unfit' should be put to death if a panel of three doctors confirmed that there was no hope of recovery. Apparently a host of 'celebrities' were quick to register their opposition to such 'wicked' proposals in the press. Among this group was the ironically named Chairman of the Eugenics Education Society, Dr Slaughter. A similar example was provided by the outrageous George Bernard Shaw[84] who in a 'notorious' speech to the Eugenics Education Society in March 1910, had seemed to advocate 'Murder by the State.' Shaw is reported to have said that eugenics 'would finally land us in an extensive use of the lethal chamber. A great many people would have to be put out of existence simply because it wastes other people's time to look after them.'[85]

Notions of eugenic euthanasia, or mercy-killing were by no means a common theme within the eugenics movement. It was a decidedly contentious subject which could not have been seriously contemplated by an organisation which until the inter-war years deemed contraception an issue too contentious with which to ally itself. Not only were mercy-killing proposals deemed repugnant and impracticable, there were strong grounds for believing that the alternatives were far more effective. Indeed eugenic concerns about the incidence of mental deficiency do appear to have some impact upon the legislative process in the first part of the twentieth century.

The rising costs of maintaining mental defectives borne by prisons and poor law authorities had elicited strong concerns. Alongside concerns about racial decay this had led to the initiation of the Royal Commission into the Care and Control of the Feeble-minded in 1904, which reported in 1908. It reported that feeble-mindedness was a hereditary affliction, that there were higher levels of fertility among the mentally impaired, and that some of these would have to be segregated for the benefit of themselves and others. Nevertheless, it was made abundantly clear that draconian measures of the sort contemplated by Goddard and others were impracticable. The Report noted:

> Doubtless it is for the welfare of the nation and of the race that the feeble-minded should be prevented from propagating their like. But a further extension of this principle might some day lead us to consider ourselves justified in putting an end to the lives of those who are distinctly obnoxious to the community; and thus we might get back to the period when capital punishment – or, as it might now be called, capital treatment – was the chief mode of preserving society. Whatever may seem justifiable in the interests of the community, in this respect, public opinion is hardly yet ripe for the application of such drastic measures.[867]

'Euthanasia' in the sense of the voluntary or non-voluntary varieties of mercy-killing failed to make any significant impact within the British medical profession before the twentieth century. Indeed discussion of these issues was negligible. For most nineteenth-century physicians 'euthanasia' was a reasonably obscure term used to refer to methods of palliative care, or more simply, making death comfortable; the wilful precipitation of a patient's death did not fall within this remit.

Notes

1 Ezekiel J. Emanuel, 'The history of euthanasia debates in the United States and Britain', *Annals of Internal Medicine*, 15 Nov. 1994, Vol, 121. No. 10, p. 795.

2 I. Van Der Sluis, 'The movement for euthanasia 1875–1975', *Janus*, Vol. 66, p. 131.

3 Voluntary Euthanasia Society Archives (VES), Contemporary Medical Archives Centre (CMAC), Wellcome Institute for the History of Medicine, Euston Road, London. CMAC/SA/VES/C.4 *Suggestions in Favour of Terminating Absolutely Hopeless Cases of Injury or Disease, being a paper by Charles E. Goddard, MD, read before the Willesden and District Medical Society, 17 May 1901*.

4 Pat Jalland, *Death in the Victorian Family* (Oxford, 1996) p. 5.

5 *Ibid.*, p. 6.

6 Peter Razzell, *The Conquest of Smallpox: The Impact of Inoculation on Smallpox* (London, 1977).

7 Thomas McKeown, *Medicine in Modern Society: Medical Planning Based on Evaluation of Medical Achievement* (London, 1965) pp. 39–58.

8 Simon Szreter, 'The importance of social intervention in Britain's mortality decline, *c.* 1850–1914: a reinterpretation of the role of public health', *Social History of Medicine*, 1, 1988, pp. 1–38.

9 Jalland, *Death in the Victorian Family*, p. 78.

10 See Bruce Fye, 'Active euthanasia: an historical survey of its conceptual origins and introduction into medical thought', *Bulletin of the History of Medicine*, 1968, pp. 493–502.

11 Roy Porter, 'Death and the doctors in Georgian England', in Ralph Houlbrook (ed.), *Death Ritual and Bereavement* (London, 1989) p. 78.

12 John Ferriar, *Medical Histories* (London, 1792) p. 10.

13 Martin Pernick, *A Calculus of Suffering* (New York, 1986) p. 22.

14 Fye, 'Active euthanasia', p. 496.

15 Jalland, *Death in the Victorian Family*, p. 81.

16 Roy Porter, *The Greatest Benefit to Mankind: A Medical History of Humanity from Antiquity to the Present* (London, 1997) p. 349.

17 Roy Porter, 'Death and the doctors', p. 90.

18 *Ibid.*, p. 91.

19 'Reviews and notices of books', *The Lancet*, 7 Jan. 1888, pp. 21–2.

20 *The Lancet*, 7 Jan. 1888, p. 22.

21 William Munk, *Euthanasia: or Medical Treatment in Aid of an Easy Death* (London, 1887) pp. 4–5.

22 *Ibid.*, p. 9.

23 *Ibid.*, p. 65.

24 *Ibid.*, p. 65.

25 *Ibid.*, pp. 66–7.

26 *Ibid.*, p. 69.

27 *Ibid.*, p. 73. My emphasis.

28 *Ibid.*, p. 81.

29 *Ibid.*, p. 5.

30 R. A. Wilson, 'A medico-literary causerie, euthanasia', *The Practitioner*, 1896, Vol. 56, pp. 631–5; *Medico-Legal Journal*, 1896, Vol. 14, pp. 103–6.

31 'May the physician ever end life?', *BMJ*, 10 Apr. 1897, p. 934.

32 Jalland, *Death in the Victorian Family*, pp. 91–2.

33 'Notes, short comments, and answers to correspondents', *The Lancet*, 18 Feb. 1899, p. 489.

34 'Euthanasia', *The Lancet*, 25 Feb. 1899, p. 532.

35 Obituaries: *BMJ*, 14 Feb. 1942, p. 241; *The Medical Officer*, 14 Feb. 1942, p. 52.

36 Goddard, *Suggestions*.

37 *Ibid.*, p. 5.

38 *On the State of Public Health, Annual Report of the Chief Medical Officer of the Ministry of Health for the Year 1927* (London, 1928) p. 99.

39 Goddard, *Suggestions*. p. 6.

40 See E. Ray Lankester, *Degeneration: A Chapter in Darwinism* (London, 1880) p. 28.

41 See Dorothy Porter, '"Enemies of the race": biologism, environmentalism, and public health in Edwardian England', *Victorian Studies*, Winter 1991,

Vol. 34, pp. 159–78.

42   Charles Darwin, *The Descent of Man, And Selection in Relation to Sex* [facsimile copy of the 1871 edition in Fireston Library, Princeton University] (Princeton, 1981) p. 168.

43   See Peter Bowler, *Charles Darwin: The Man and his Influence*, (Cambridge, 1996) p. 197; Charles Darwin, *The Descent of Man*, pp. 168–9.

44   Although the term was not introduced until 1883 Galton had first published his eugenic ideas in 1865 in a two-part article for *Macmillan's Magazine*. This was subsequently expanded into a book published in 1869 entitled *Hereditary Genius*.

45   Francis Galton, 'Eugenics, Its sefinition, scope and aims', Sociological Papers I (1905) 45, extract cited in C. P. Blacker, *Eugenics in Retrospect and Prospect*, The Galton Lecture 1945, delivered on 16 Feb., 1945 at Manson House, London. (London, 1950) p. 21.

46   David Barker, 'How to curb the fertility of the unfit: the feeble-minded in Edwardian Britain', *Oxford Review of Education*, Vol. 9, No. 3, 1983.

47   Richard Soloway, *Demography and Degeneration* (Chapel Hill, 1990) p. 20.

48   John Berry Haycraft, *Darwinism and Race Progress* (London, 1895).

49   *Ibid.*, p. 86.

50   *Ibid.*, p. 88.

51   Arnold White, *The Problems of a Great City* (London, 1887).

52   *Ibid.*, pp. 28–30.

53   Martin S. Pernick, *The Black Stork: Eugenics and the Death of Defectives Babies in American Medicine and Motion Pictures Since 1915* (New York, Oxford, 1996).

54   F. H. Bradley, 'Some remarks on punishment', *International Journal of Ethics*, April 1894.

55   *Ibid.*, pp. 281–2.

56   Founded in 1907.

57   Founded in 1935.

58   Goddard, *Suggestions*, p. 8.

59   *Ibid.*

60   *Ibid.*, pp. 8–9.

61   Edward Renvoize, 'The Association of Medical Officers of Asylums and Hospitals for the Insane, the Medico-Psychological Association and their Presidents', in Hugh Freeman and German Berrios (eds), *150 Years of British Psychiatry* (London, 1991) p. 70.

62   Lockhart Robertson (1867), Sir James Coxe (1872) and Rayner (1884).

63   Renvoize, 'Association', p. 61.

64   Appendix A to *Fifth Report of the Board of Control*, p. 1.

65   W. F. Bynum, Roy Porter, and Michael Shepherd (eds), *The Anatomy of Madness: Essays in the History of Psychiatry*, Vol. 3 (London, 1988) p. 4.

66   Goddard, *Suggestions*, p. 12.

67   Robert Rentoul, *Race Culture or Race Suicide? A Plea for the Unborn* (London, 1906).

68   G. R. Searle, *Eugenics and Politics, 1900–1914* (Leyden, 1976) p. 93.

69   Rentoul, *Race Culture*, p. 46.

70   *Ibid.*, pp. 2–3.

71   *Ibid.*, pp. 9–10.

72   *Ibid.*, p. 42.

73 *Ibid.*
74 *Ibid.*, p. 36.
75 *Ibid.*, pp. 170–1.
76 Goddard, *Suggestions*, p. 5.
77 Robert Saunby, *Medical Ethics: A Guide to Professional Conduct* (1902).
78 See Michael Bliss, *William Osler: A Life in Medicine* (Oxford, 1999) pp. 321–8.
79 *BMJ*, 18 Mar. 1905, p. 618.
80 *BMJ*, 17 Mar. 1906, p. 638.
81 *Ibid.*
82 *Ibid.*, p. 818.
83 *Ibid.*, pp. 638–9.
84 Shaw was a future member of the Voluntary Euthanasia (Legalisation) Society, as well as being a member of the Eugenics Education Society.
85 Archives of the Eugenics Society, Contemporary Medical Archives Centre, Euston Road, London SA/EUG NI,3,4, press cuttings 11 Nov. 1909–10 May 1910. *Daily Express*, 4 Mar. 1909. Shaw's speech received considerable coverage in no less than fourteen daily newspapers.
86 Art. 9 The Control of the Feeble-Minded, Report of the Royal Commission on the Care and Control of the Feeble-minded [Cmd. 4202], 1908, cited in *Quarterly Review*, Vol. 210, Jan.–Apr., 1909, p. 174.

3

The missing link: discussion of mercy-killing 1910–30

Existing accounts of the British euthanasia movement are rather episodic. They portray a brief but concerted debate in the 1870s, followed by a trickle of articles up to 1906, and then a period of comparative silence until the 1930s.[1] This is not entirely inaccurate. It was only in the 1930s that the euthanasia debate really erupted, becoming the focus of sustained discussion for both the medical profession and the broader intellectual population. Yet one might have assumed that with large numbers of casualties on the battlefield and limited supplies of palliative drugs the question of mercy-killing would have become a more pressing practical consideration during the course of the First World War.

As early as 1873, Lionel Tollemache had noted that the case for euthanasia was supported by the fact that some people would have to endure the 'hardest fate of all', that of a mortally wounded soldier who wants to die 'but whose wounds are laboriously tended; so that by an ingenious cruelty he is kept suffering, against nature, and against his own will'.[2] The poet Charles Sorley remarked upon the 'relief' felt when 'the bullet or bomb that made man an animal É made the animal a corpse'.[3] Doctors were also forced to prioritise treatment of patients who could be returned quickly and efficiently to the war effort rather than concentrate their energies on patients who stood little chance of survival.[4] Despite this, there is no indication that mercy-killing in these circumstances received any serious consideration. Of course it is possible that it was practised, but it seems likely that a rifle shot from a fellow soldier rather than a lethal injection of scarce narcotics would have been the preferred method.

As we have seen discussion of mercy-killing among the medical profession was fairly negligible. The alleged quietude of this intervening period is therefore plausible. It is not unreasonable to suppose that an already muted discussion would have paled into insignificance while the Great War was in progress, culling huge numbers of young men, or in its aftermath, while the flu epidemic was ravaging the population.[5] Indeed, a notable feature of this period is the continuing absence of discussion about euthanasia among medics. Only a handful of articles appeared in the medical press, all dealing with the question in the most perfunctory fashion.[6] However, a close examination of the period indicates that discussion of particular forms of mercy-killing did persist. This fragmented discussion took place in a number of rather diverse publications and was concerned primarily with the home front rather than the theatre of war. The debate was not particularly widespread nor was it intense. It was rather disjointed and lacked the coherence of preceding and succeeding eras, but to ignore these texts would impoverish the historical record of the British euthanasia debate. It would also neglect the development of important themes which recur after 1930.

By the second decade of the twentieth century, the classical notion of euthanasia seems to have given way to the concept of mercy-killing.[7] Before the First World War, this was usually rejected on grounds of the inaccuracy of medical diagnoses, and because it contravened the edicts of the Hippocratic Oath.[8] Thereafter discussion gradually became more frequent and views more varied. Despite the eclipse of euthanasia in the classical sense, the concept continued to embrace two distinct meanings: mercy-killing for the *compos mentis*, and non-voluntary mercy-killing for the mentally defective. As the previous chapter indicated, there has been a tendency for discussion of the former practice to bleed into a discussion of the latter. However, between the wars there was a more overt and deliberate focus on the non-voluntary aspect, as a distinct proposal in its own right. At this time eugenic ideas were enjoying something of a resurgence[9] and seem to have fed into discussion of mercy-killing, a trend which enjoyed a degree of international currency.[10]

Proposals for the non-voluntary killing of mental defectives were motivated by a number of factors. At one level there was genuine concern that the lives of the mentally defective were bereft of happiness and were often characterised by pronounced suffering which ought to be relieved. Among particular eugenicists, however, there was a tendency to consider forms of life which diverged from a narrowly defined ideal as distinctly undesirable, regardless of the individual's potential to enjoy life. Allied to this were assessments of the opportunity costs of maintaining defectives; a crude calculus of an individual's net contribution or cost to society as a whole. According to this view, it was the aggregate well-being of society rather than the individual which should predominate if these interests were not congruent with one another. At this time discussion of mercy-killing became part of a discussion about the costs of medical care and, in particular, psychiatric care. Scarcity of resources created an economic debate about the sums spent on dealing with marginal figures in society, this occasionally elicited rather crude proposals for disposing of mental defectives.

Ultimately, proposals for non-voluntary euthanasia were rejected in Britain. Politically, they were unacceptable, and eugenically the alternatives were considered to be more effective. By 1931 proposals for the mercy killing of the *non compos mentis* had been almost entirely supplanted by a concerted focus on voluntary euthanasia for the terminally ill. These proposals were themselves partly a function of changes in attitudes to death engendered by the First World War. They would also succeed in arousing a far greater degree of popular support. Nevertheless, the euthanasia debate after 1930 would retain an identifiable stream of opinion which sought to extend euthanasia to defectives, and it seems important, therefore, to trace its foundations and motivations. Indeed, despite the prevalence of slippery-slope arguments throughout the history of the euthanasia movement, we find that during the 1920s proposals for voluntary euthanasia tended to be distilled from proposals of non-voluntary euthanasia rather than the more common assumption that proposals of voluntary euthanasia lead to the advocacy of non-voluntary euthanasia.

The First World War claimed the lives of approximately three-quarters of a million Britons. This accounted for some 7 per cent of the male population of England and Wales between the ages of fifteen and forty-nine in 1911.[11] Some 30.58 per cent of all men aged twenty to twenty-four in 1914 were killed and 28.15 per cent of those aged thirteen to nineteen.[12] Because the war losses were so pronounced in this age category, the notion of a 'lost generation' gained considerable currency. This was considered to have a strong qualitative as well as quantitative dimension. In contrast to commentators such as Herbert Spencer, who had extolled the beneficial effects of war from the perspective of racial improvement in primitive societies, it was generally recognised that among highly civilised societies, war tended to be counter-selective. From the start of the war, the *Eugenics Review* had lamented the fact that mentally and physically superior individuals were the first to volunteer for active service. Modern warfare was said to be 'almost entirely dysgenic'.[13] Educated members of the upper classes constituted a significant proportion of the first wave of casualties, prompting the view that the country was losing its most able future leaders. This was compounded by the fact that particular professions were protected. Manual labourers engaged in mining or engineering work were prevented from enlisting. In addition, the poor physical condition of many of the Edwardian working classes ensured a much higher rejection rate among this group. Over 40 per cent of men in the professional classes joined the armed forces between 1914 and 1916, compared with only 25 per cent of miners.[14] Britain's dependence on a volunteer army led many eugenists to the conclusion that racially, Britain would suffer more than other countries.[15] Although such a policy was more likely to ensure 'victory' and 'national prestige' the effect in racial terms was thought to be 'injurious', it might even be 'disastrous'. The 'cream of the race' would be taken and the 'skimmed milk' would be left.[16]

It was for these reasons that Leonard Darwin, the President of the Eugenics Society, became an early advocate of conscription. In his view this would ensure that casualty lists would approximate more closely 'a random sample of the population'.[17] Before the adoption of conscription in 1916, it had seemed impossible to 'avoid the disproportionate loss of the most "chivalrous, virile and courageous young men"'.[18] In the course of his Presidential Address to the Annual General Meeting of the Eugenics Society in 1915, Darwin remarked that Britain's military system seemed to be so designed as to protect the 'defective in mind or body' from being shot at. The eugenically 'unfit' were kept at home and unfortunately propagated a stock which would 'deteriorate the natural qualities of the coming generations'.[19] Even before the war, population growth had begun to slow, ensuring that Britain's population was an ageing one. In 1841 almost half of the population was under the age of twenty, by 1911 this had shrunk to less than a third.[20] The perceived consequence was a watering down of Britain's racial vitality. Eugenist Caleb Saleeby remarked that if a nation relied upon its 'trash' rather than its 'treasure' to do the fighting, 'war might be defended as a dreadful purgative of nations – God's medicine for the human race, as Treitschke calls it'.[21]

Similar concerns were evident amongst particular psychiatrists. In a Presidential Address entitled 'War and the Burden of Insanity', delivered to the seventy-seventh annual meeting of the Medico-Psychological Association in 1918, John Keay, MD, FRCPE, Lt Col RAMC, noted that biologically war was counter-selective.[22] Like Darwin, he observed that the voluntary system of military service which had operated during the first two years of the war had led to a deterioration of the racial stock. Even with the advent of compulsory military service, the 'young', 'strong' and 'healthy' were selected to face the grave risk of 'death or disablement'. The 'old', 'feeble' and 'unfit' on the other hand were 'carefully preserved' along with the clergy, inmates of asylums and Members of Parliament. This was considered to be 'enough to make a eugenist scream'.[23]

Keay's address provides a classic example of the fusion of eugenic and economic arguments. Because of the huge expenditure necessitated by the exigencies of war it was suggested that there would need to be considerable fiscal belt-tightening. This necessity for thriftiness and economy also extended to the asylum. Keay noted that the cost of maintaining asylums in England, Scotland and Wales amounted to an annual sum of £4.6 million. Although these figures were comparatively small alongside wartime expenditure, opportunity costs in military terms were rehearsed in some detail. These sums would be sufficient to add to the Navy 'two super-dreadnoughts, built, armed, and equipped, every year'.[24]

Although he had eloquently outlined the way in which money was being wasted on unproductive policies, Keay was not an advocate of non-voluntary euthanasia. Despite regarding the chronically insane as the most 'helpless and pitiable class ... bereft for their lives of the priceless possessions of health and personal liberty', he stated quite clearly that no reduction in expenditure which necessitated an adverse shift in their 'conditions of life would be tolerated for a moment by the ratepayers of this country'. Rather than cutting the maintenance costs of the 'hopelessly and incurably insane' the proposed reduction in expenditure was to be achieved by 'limiting their number'.[25] It was the prevention of insanity with which Keay's address was principally concerned. This was indeed the general thrust of eugenic policy during this period.

The pronatalist schemes advocated since the late nineteenth century were considered increasingly incapable of dealing with the scale of the racial problem which war was believed to have unleashed. In this atmosphere, we can see the reserve with which eugenists had advanced negative eugenic policies before 1914, steadily giving way to the advocacy of restrictive policies. Heightened concerns about the incidence of mental deficiency were particularly evident at this time, and gave rise to developments such as the Eugenics Society's campaign for voluntary sterilisation. Indeed, a great deal of secondary literature has been devoted to the attempts to legalise sterilisation for the mentally defective.[26] But these efforts were concerned primarily with those whose mental incapacity was comparatively slight. They pertained to the 'feeble-minded', rather than the category of so-called 'low-grade' defectives: the 'imbeciles' and 'idiots'. Too often, discussion of eugenics between the wars fails to differentiate between different grades of mental capacity.[27] While the term 'feeble-minded' was occasionally used in a generic sense, to denote all grades of defect, it actually had a more precise definition referring to the mildest form of mental defect. Members of this class were said to be capable of making 'tolerable' progress at elementary school. They were able to read and write, and do simple arithmetic. They could undertake basic and routine work with the minimum of supervision and were able to earn a living given the appropriate occupation and 'treated with a little indulgence and some oversight'. Yet, they were incapable of budgeting in order to provide for themselves. They were unable to plan for the future and could not 'co-ordinate their conduct in such a way as to enable them to maintain an existence independently of outside supervision'.[28]

Professor R. J. A. Berry, an authority on mental deficiency, described the feeble-minded as similar in appearance to the ordinary members of society, but whose 'undeveloped brain' made them 'a menace to the community'. Their standards of moral conduct, particularly sexual, were considered to be highly deficient. A feeble-minded individual was deemed to have deficient 'prudence' and 'foresight'. They tended to breed 'freely', and 'far too frequently' were 'allowed to survive and thrive through misguided activities of charitable organisations who, in defiance of all natural law, encourage the survival of the unfit'.[29]

Below the feeble-minded in terms of defect were the 'imbeciles', the 'medium-grade aments'. These individuals were capable of reading and spelling monosyllabic words. They were able to count upon their fingers, 'tell their name ... recognize and name common objects.' The less afflicted of the class were able to perform simple tasks, and to help in domestic chores if told precisely what to do. They were also capable of washing, dressing and feeding themselves if supervised. However, the capacity of the 'medium-grade imbecile' to engage in employment was significantly less than that of the 'feeble-minded'. He was incapable of performing any task 'without oversight; whilst the *lowest grade* approximate to the idiots, and are incapable of any useful work'. None of them were deemed capable of earning sufficient remuneration to 'pay for their keep'.[30]

The lowest grade of defective was the 'idiot', the most distinguishing characteristic of which was an inability to comprehend or avoid 'physical dangers which threaten existence'. Idiots were considered incapable of undertaking any 'useful task'. They were unable to wash or dress themselves and in most cases were monosyllabic. Among the most 'profound' cases there was a 'lack of the fundamental organic instincts, no power of attention, and a complete incapacity for being taught'.[31] It is the contention of this chapter that the increasingly pronounced, negative bent of eugenics between the wars facilitated discussion of mercy-killing for the more severe cases of mental defect. This is a debate which has been rather overlooked by the secondary literature on eugenics.

Of course non-voluntary euthanasia was not the most readily advocated tool of negative eugenics, and it comes as little surprise to learn than other practices tended to be favoured. The President of the Eugenics Education Society, Major Leonard Darwin, was quite categorical in ruling out eugenic mercy-killing. His text of 1926 text entitled *The Need For Eugenic Reform*[32] considered four mechanisms for the elimination of mental defect, these were: segregation, sterilisation, conception control and the 'lethal chamber'. Of these, killing of the 'unfit' was deemed unacceptable. Darwin argued that the association of 'murder' with social progress might produce an increase in the murder rate, it would cause considerable distress for those who might be 'eliminated' and also for those whose 'beloved' relatives might fall within the scope of such a programme. Although the racial effects of such a policy were potentially beneficial, the alternatives were considered to be more humane. They would also be more readily adopted and consequently, would prove to be a more effective tool of racial improvement. Darwin was quite explicit on this issue, noting that 'scientific baby murder' could not be tolerated. Eugenic reform should never be effected through the 'agency of the death rate ... but only through that of the birth rate'.[33]

The matter was also discussed by the eminent neurologist and eugenist, A. F. Tredgold, in the fourth edition of his classic textbook, *Mental Deficiency: Amentia*. Tredgold, who was the leading authority on mental defect and had been an expert witness before the Royal Commission on the Care and Control of the Feeble-minded of 1908, discussed the idea of a lethal chamber for those with severe mental defect but ruled it out as impracticable; a position which he would later reverse.[34] He remarked that society had to recognise that mental defectives existed, and 'must be allowed to exist, and the questions before us are as to the way in which the State can best deal with them, and the manner in which it can prevent their procreation'.[35] He conceded that there were strong arguments both for and against mercy-killing and suggested that society would not necessarily be 'unjustified' in adopting such a measure as a 'self-defence' mechanism for 'ridding itself of its anti-social constituents', but public opinion was such that this proposal could not be contemplated at the present juncture.

The First World War has often been depicted as the eugenists' worst nightmare, because it killed off the most 'fit' leaving an alleged legion of the 'unfit' to propagate the stock.[36] But the 'imbeciles' and 'idiots' who were necessarily left behind in the asylums certainly did not enjoy a pampered existence. If the counter-selectivity of modern society had sponsored the survival of the 'worst' elements of society, the war did much to relieve these constraints exposing the unfortunates of the asylum to conditions which many did not survive. The substantial increase in the death rate on the home front is invariably glossed over in accounts of the human toll of the First World War. Yet, it is clear that prioritisation of human resources and rationing of food had grave consequences for the 'incompetent'. This has been entirely omitted from accounts of British eugenics.

By 1917 the rise in the asylum death rate had reached such proportions that the Board of Control decided to appoint a Committee to visit the institutions where the death rate had been most acute in order to ascertain the causes and to provide suggestions for the resolution of these problems.[37] For half a century prior to 1915 the death rate in asylums had registered a small but sustained decline. The years 1909–14 had registered an average death rate of 9.7 per cent of the daily average number of residents. The following year the death rate rose to 12.1 per cent; a figure not reached since 1860.[38] During 1917 the figure had risen to 17.6 per cent. The disparity between the death returns for the years 1916–17 and the last year of the pre-war period indicated that the sharp rise in mortality levels was a function of the 'disproportionate' increase in the number of deaths from 'tuberculosis, senility (including arteriosclerosis), pneumonia, dysentery, and enteric fever'.[39] Having visited twenty-six institutions the commissioners came to the conclusion that in most cases, the rise in the number of deaths was due solely to war conditions. This included, the 'unavoidable reduction in quantity, and deterioration in quality of the food supplied to patients'.[40] This had raised levels of sickness and mortality 'amongst patients in institutions for the insane and defective'.[40]

Even if the dietary provisions had been normal, there would still have been a 'considerable rise over pre-war death rates due to other war conditions'.[42] These included the greater age and lower physical condition of patients admitted to asylums after 1914. Fewer men between the ages of 18 and 41 had been sent to asylums, being admitted only if they were 'physically unfit for military service'.[43] The demand for female labour in factories meant that many 'weaklings could no longer be looked after in their own houses'.[44] The closure of workhouses led to an increase in the number of patients admitted to asylums suffering from senility. The closure of particular asylums for war hospital purposes led to a degree of redistribution from asylum to asylum, and this aided the introduction of disease and the spread of epidemics in institutions hitherto unaffected.

The fact that a number of asylums were closed in order to provide space for war hospitals led to overcrowding, which combined with bad ventilation (caused by the necessity of masking windows by curtains to comply with lighting restrictions) exacerbated problems in cases of infectious disease 'especially phthisis'. Impairments in staff efficiency 'incident upon decreased numbers, untrained character of substitutes, and frequent changes' resulted in a decline in cleanliness.[45] Because a considerable proportion of the wartime asylum staff were untrained, there was a tendency to detect illness only in its more advanced forms. Sick and infectious patients were also inadequately segregated, which aided the spread of dysenteric and tubercular diseases. This was compounded by the lack of personal cleanliness. Frequent handling of food with dirty hands, re-wearing of soiled underclothing, and inappropriate handling of foul linen, all increased the potential for spreading disease. In the light of these revelations, the comments of Keay, Tredgold and Darwin may be interpreted as a recognition that the accidental rise in the death rate among the eugenically undesirable was not a policy which could be effected intentionally in peacetime.

Others were less restrained. In 1928 a remarkable essay on the 'Right to die' appeared in a volume entitled *Democracy on Trial*,[46] by the little-known F. A. W. Gisborne.The premise of this book was that democracy was distinctly undesirable, because it resulted in 'continual change and insecurity, faction and social discord'.[47] This was perhaps not such an unusual premise bearing in mind the politically unstable environment of Europe between the wars. 'Good government' was considered infinitely preferable to an inherently unstable system of popular government, and Gisborne appears to have favoured the installation of a non-elected expertocracy. Precisely what bearing such proposals had upon the 'Right to die' is not immediately apparent. Yet, if we probe Gisborne's remarks more carefully, we find that his mercy-killing proposals were underpinned by eugenic and economic rationales and appear to have been concerned with the 'Right to kill' as well as the 'Right to die'.

Gisborne noted that in modern society there was a tendency to prolong life for its own sake, even when accompanied by intractable and terminal suffering. There was also an inclination 'to pamper weaklings, to neglect the claims of the deserving, and to lavish favours on the unworthy'.[48] Evidently, he was unfamiliar with the Board of Control reports. Referring to an eminent ecclesiastic who had predicted that society would soon kill 'more freely but mercifully', he suggested that the sooner this prophecy was realised with regard to 'physical, mental and moral incurables ... the better'. He proposed the painless removal of cases of 'hopeless insanity'. He argued that in the interests of society it was necessary to remove the 'diseased twig' from the 'tree of life', in order to prevent the spread of infection to the 'other limbs'.[49] He wished to include sufferers of senility, and mental defectives more broadly. The prevailing mechanisms for treating both the mild and extreme forms of mental disease were considered atrocious. They were 'permeated with false sentiment and false humanity'. The 'feeble-minded' were permitted to 'roam at large, preying on the healthy, and polluting the stream of life'. Instead, they should be permanently institutionalised. In such an environment they might lead 'innocent' lives, entailing a modicum of happiness and usefulness. The 'hopeless imbecile' on the other hand was deemed to require a far more draconian approach. To prolong the life of these individuals was 'sheer cruelty'. Such arguments indicate a fusion of humanitarian and eugenic concerns, but also the belief that 'idiots' and 'imbeciles' were an insult to human dignity.

In applying the concept of the sanctity of human life to the 'mindless', immeasurable harm was said to arise. Gisborne cited the example of a woman who had died leaving behind two children. The daughter was fit and healthy, but the son was afflicted by 'a most revolting kind of imbecility'. Prior to her mother's death, the daughter had pledged that she would look after her brother for the span of his natural life. Despite the fact that he lived to the age of sixty-three, the daughter kept her promise. As a result the 'dead mind' was 'chained' to that of the daughter and prevented her from living a useful or happy life. Because of a 'false conception of her duty', she inflicted on herself the companionship of a wretched gibbering creature, whose life should have been gently extinguished as soon as it became certain that there was no hope of cure'.[50] Such 'self-sacrifice' was considered to be 'repugnant' to 'reason' and 'humanity'.

Gisborne's proposals were also suffused with a strong economic rationale. It was noted that an enormous waste of 'money, service and philanthropic energy' was involved in a system in which 'mere existence' seemed to be valued more highly than 'happiness and usefulness'. He remarked that in a 'densely populated country' such as England, the struggle for subsistence was becoming increasingly 'desperate'. This was not without foundation. Perhaps the most significant feature of the social fabric between the wars was the problem of mass unemployment. The series of acts which had been passed in order to provide benefit over and above that accounted for under the insurance scheme, ensured that the financial burden was far from negligible. In addition to this, attention was drawn to the heavy burden imposed upon the healthy members of the populace by sustaining the large number of asylums, nursing homes, prisons and hospitals for incurables which threatened to become unbearable. Large numbers of individuals were also required to tend to the needs of the 'aged' and 'chronic invalids'.[51]

It was suggested that an inherent feature of the democratic system was that parties attempted to attract the support of voters by offering various enticements. While this was invariably successful in electoral terms, it ensured that a considerable financial burden was thrust upon the 'wealth-reproducing classes' for the purpose of maintaining 'a host of physical and mental weaklings'. Ultimately, this burden would prove to be too heavy to bear. No community could sponsor 'idleness' in perpetuity; such a policy was 'scarcely conducive to racial improvement'.[52]

The crux of Gisborne's book centred on the notion that 'long life' was not in itself desirable. '[M]ental and physical vigour' allied with 'happiness' and 'usefulness' were the prerequisites for worthwhile life. Once they had departed, the sooner the 'vital flame' was put out, the 'better'. The prolongation of worthless life was deemed 'cruel and unprofitable'. This utopian future world, would be one in which 'eugenic ideals' prevailed. This would involve the regulation of both birth and death. It would be considered the 'deepest of sins' to deliver a 'human being into a world with a stone round its neck'. Individuals would enter life free from 'cruel transmitted infirmities' and 'endowed with all the physical, mental and moral qualities necessary to happiness and the full performance of social duties'. When, as a result of 'disease, accident or age', life became burdensome to the individual and others, life would be laid down.[53]

Between the wars, the subject of mental deficiency had indeed become the focus of renewed and sustained concern.[54] This was evidenced most clearly by the establishment of the Inter-departmental Committee on Mental Deficiency which reported in 1929. The Committee had been established in 1924 with the purpose of ascertaining the extent of mental deficiency in England and Wales and assessing the degree to which the provisions of the Mental Deficiency Act of 1913 were operating effectively. The Wood Report,[55] as it was more commonly known, suggested that the incidence of mental deficiency had increased quite markedly since the Royal Commission on the Care and Control of the Feeble-minded of 1908.

The chief investigator of the Committee was Dr E. O. Lewis, who was also a member of the Eugenics Society. While the Report of 1908 had recorded that 4.6 per thousand population suffered from mental defect, Lewis's statistics for 1928 revealed that this had risen to 0.56 per thousand. The Committee conceded that such a marked increase might be attributable, in part, to Lewis's improved techniques of ascertainment. In addition to the returns from asylums, prisons and other institutions, which had been employed in the 1908 Report, Lewis also conducted his own mental tests on schoolchildren referred to him by teachers on the basis of alleged feeble-mindedness. Nevertheless, the Committee was quite resolute in its view that the incidence of mental deficiency had been subject to a genuine and pronounced increase. As we saw in our considera-tion of Gisborne, his proposals for dealing with mental deficiency contained a strong component of fiscal reasoning. Similar senti-ments were also evident with regard to the Wood Report. The social-biologist, Lancelot Hogben, had pointed out 'that if all the feeble-minded were placed in institutions, the cost in 1929–30 would have been about 12 million pounds – about one-tenth of Britain's armaments expenditure that year'.[56]

Historians have tended to emphasise the Report's claim that high-grade mental deficiency was concentrated among families whose intelligence was below the norm, whereas pronounced, or low-grade defectives were distributed 'indiscriminately in all social strata'.[57] Attention has also been focused on the suggestion that lurking behind the 340,000 or so people who were actually certifi-able as mentally defective, there was a significantly larger group of 'sub-cultural' relatives.[58] It was believed that this Social Problem Group accounted for as much as 10 per cent of the population. The Report noted that 'mental deficiency', 'physical inefficiency', 'chronic pauperism' and 'recidivism' were all intimately related and constituted 'one of the major social problems which a civilised community may be called upon to solve'.[59] Claims of this nature had profound implications for the eugenics movement. They were instrumental in providing the basis for the campaign to legalise voluntary sterilisation for mental defectives, which had become the 'leading ideological edge' of the eugenics movement by the late 1920s.[60] Nevertheless, while 'imbecility' and 'idiocy' were not considered to pose the same social problems as 'feeble-minded-ness',[61] the investigation had 'revealed twice as many lower-grade defectives as did that of the Royal Commission twenty years previ-ously'. The ratio of different grades to each other was also believed to have remained the same.[62] These factors were not unimportant with regard to the mercy-killing debate between the wars.

While most experts in the field of mental deficiency felt unable to support the mercy-killing of hopeless defectives, there were occasional exceptions. Professor Richard J. A. Berry, who after a distinguished career in Australia in the fields of anatomy and mental deficiency returned to Britain in 1930 to be become director of medical services at the Stoke Park Colony for mental defectives at Stapleton, Bristol provides a case in point.[63] Berry was famed for having pioneered research into the correlation of cerebral amentia and abnormal head size.[64] Following his return to England, he wasted little time in making strident pronouncements which caused the Eugenics Society considerable embarrassment.

In 1930 the *Eugenics Review* made reference to Berry's proposal for a 'lethal chamber, under State control', designed for the 'painless extermination' of low-grade defectives. The *Review* remarked upon the need to restrain the 'more enthusiastic advocates' of negative eugenics. Dr Berry's proposal had apparently provoked a 'storm of protest' and it was considered deeply unfortunate that it had been made. His prescription of a 'lethal chamber' would incur 'almost insuperable legal and practical difficulties'. Moreover, it was suggested that the eradication of the 'genetically defective' could be accomplished by a 'judicious combination' of sterilisation and segregation. The *Eugenics Review* concluded that '[e]xtreme proposals' were always counter-productive, and it was hoped that eugenics would not 'run the risk of being regarded as anything other than it is – a reasonable, organic development of the policy of public health'.[65]

This was a strong condemnation of Berry's proposals and it is certainly true that proposals of this nature had never resembled anything like an orthodox view among the members of the Eugenics Society. However, the *Review* also noted that Berry's prescription had 'provoked a rather surprising amount of support'. Attention was also drawn to a review of a German publication which had dealt with a similar issue. This book alluded to a survey conducted by Ewald Meltzer, director of the Katharinehof asylum at Grosshennersdorf in Saxony, Germany.[66] Meltzer had asked '200 parents of aments whether they would be willing to have their children destroyed: 162 replied, and 73 per cent of them said yes.' It should be pointed out that Meltzer was in fact a strong critic of such a policy. Indeed, his book in which this study was contained, had been published as a response to a tract of 1920 by Professor Karl Binding and Professor Alfred Hoche,[67] entitled *Permission for the Destruction of Worthless Life, its Extent and Form.*[68] This text, like those we have examined in a British context, had been written against the backdrop of economic hardship and a drive for economy in the aftermath of the First World War. As in Britain, prioritisation of scarce resources was already a reality, causing significant increases in levels of asylum mortality. This text posed the question of whether there was human life which had 'so far forfeited the character of something entitled to enjoy the protection of the law, that its prolongation' represented a 'perpetual loss of value, both for its bearer and for society as a whole'.[69]

The text identified three categories of potential recipients of euthanasia. The first proposal was for the voluntary euthanasia of the terminally-ill or wounded patients. The second category included those patients who had lost consciousness and consequently were unable to make their own decision about life or death. In such cases it was proposed to have a third party anticipate their wishes for them. The final category was concerned with 'incurable idiots', individuals who were not of the 'slightest use', but provided an enormous burden, absorbing resources which might be employed more usefully in the task of national regeneration. In a similar fashion to British eugenists such as Keay, economic costs in terms of foodstuffs, clothing, heating and the wages of those working in asylums were all rehearsed in detail. As these 'ballast existences' allegedly lacked self-awareness and possessed no 'will to live', it was considered legitimate to terminate their lives. Binding and Hoche argued that they represented a 'travesty of real human beings, occasioning disgust in anyone who encounters them'.[70] It was suggested that society had ceased to regard the 'state organism as a whole' replete with 'its own laws and requirements' in the same way that doctors know a 'self-contained organism' abandons and rejects 'individual parts' which had become 'worthless or damaging'.[71]

Such discussion, emanating from the psychiatric profession of Weimar Germany, is often identified as providing the long-term foundations upon which the Nazi euthanasia programme was built. This was a programme which between 1939 and 1945 was responsible for the extermination of approximately 100,000 liberally defined 'defectives'. But, without any pretensions to sensationalism, we should not let these events detract from the fact that mercy-killing discussions in the two respective countries were, occasionally, interchangeable. The texts of Berry or Gisborne would not have been out of place alongside that of Binding and Hoche. This is certainly not to suggest that Britain was merely lacking the political will to implement a Nazi-style euthanasia programme. Nevertheless, it does seem appropriate to temper the widespread view that the euthanasia debate in Germany was such a case apart. Discussion of the Nazi policy of killing mental defectives frequently uses the term euthanasia only in inverted commas. The logic of this is to indicate that the programme of 1939–45 diverged so radically from modern-day notions of euthanasia that there is a need to demarcate these very different concepts in order to avoid confusion. It should be stressed, however, that between the wars in both Great Britain and Germany euthanasia embraced both notions. If we wish to avoid a distortion of the historical record, we should be decidedly cautious of projecting normative notions of euthanasia on to the debate which took place at this time.

In precisely the same way that Binding and Hoche advocated both voluntary euthanasia and non-voluntary euthanasia for mental defectives, so did Gisborne. Indeed, as we have noted in previous chapters, there has been a tendency for these proposals to run into one another. Gisborne suggested that victims of incurable physical disease should be injected with strong opiates to curtail life. The procedure would be conducted by at least two physicians who would face no legal censure. He remarked that there was an unfortunate and widespread inclination 'to be kind only to be cruel, to prolong suffering instead of bestowing the only possible relief'.[72] Evidently he put considerable store in the notion of medical paternalism, for he stated that the patient's permission would not be sought and the patient's relatives would not be asked for their opinion. The matter should be left entirely in the hands of 'medical experts', as this would ensure that there would be 'no cause for after regrets'.[73] He lamented what he saw as the 'disease known as sentimentalism' and the 'infinite harm' which was being brought about by the disparity between 'benevolence' and 'judgement and common sense'. Like Tollemache and Williams before him, Gisborne was keen to draw attention to the hypocrisy of the notion of the sanctity of human life, which he believed was untenable in a modern world punctuated by war and violent revolution. He

remarked that '[h]ardly any educated people' clung to the 'mediae-
val superstition that the man who, after all, has injured no one, but
possibly conferred a real service on his relations by retiring voluntarily from the world, was guilty of the crime of self-murder'.[74]
Indeed, the prevalence of suicide was regarded as an indication of
civilisation. It was common in classical antiquity, where a voluntary
death was 'frequently esteemed as an honourable death'. Among
the 'lowest savages' the practice was almost entirely unheard of,
being most common among the 'highly civilised peoples'. Of the
European nations, the 'Teutonic and the Scandinavian' countries
had the highest suicide rates, and those territories bordering the
Mediterranean the lowest.[75] In particular cases suicide was considered to be of benefit to the person concerned, to his relatives and to
society generally.[76]

Throughout preceding chapters we have observed that the
Christian concept of the sanctity of human life has been subject to
persistent objection. Between the wars this trend gained momen-
tum. War demonstrated how easily and cheaply human life could
be dispensed with. The war effort had also received almost unani-
mous ecclesiastical support. 'A favourite text for memorials was
John 15.13: "Greater love hath no man than this, that a man lay
down his life for his friends."'[77]

The First World War seems to have been instrumental in securing the ideal climate for reappraising ethical precepts concerning
the sanctity of human life and the extent to which it was deemed
acceptable to interfere with divine providence. The sheer scale of
human loss combined with the suddenness and anonymity of so
many deaths at the front precluded the exercise of traditional
Christian burial and profoundly affected the experience of death
within the family. It also seems to have done much to displace the
already weakened notion of the Christian 'good death'.

During the course of the nineteenth century an 'elaborate
etiquette of mourning' had developed, but during the war the sheer
number of casualties ensured that 'full mourning became exceptional'.[78] Indeed, it has been suggested that the 'war largely
destroyed the remaining Victorian spiritual resources which had
enabled individuals and families to perceive positive meanings in
the death of loved ones. The meaning of life and the meaning of
death were both transformed by the Great War.'[79] The combination
of evolutionary thought, biblical criticism and views of a compas-

sionate God had already brought into question the resolute doctrines of heaven and hell which had prevailed until the mid-nineteenth century. In 1929, in the preface to the *Legend of Hell*, Percy Dearmer remarked that although it remained in popular consciousness, the doctrine of hell and everlasting torment had been abandoned by most theologians as 'clearly revolting to modern conscience'.[80]

Before the outbreak of war, church membership had registered an increase both in absolute terms and relative to population size, but during the war, the latter of these two phenomenon was reversed. Although the combined membership of the Catholic and Protestant churches remained numerically robust at around eight million for the period 1914–45, this masked what has been described as the 'decline of organised religion, judged both in terms of the allegiance and membership of the Christian churches and their role as arbiters of public conventions and private morality'.[81] As Mews has suggested, 'The nation under arms presented a quite extraordinary challenge which chaplains had tried to meet, but it had to be ruefully admitted that their ministry had been appreciated only by a minority; services had not been as popular as concerts.'[82]

After the war there were pan-denominational efforts to broaden religious appeal. These took a variety of different forms, but within the Church of England, we can identify several prominent clerics who identified the need for the Church to modify its stance on particular matters of practical ethics. To some extent this was a coming to terms with particular secular social trends such as the increased use of contraceptive devices. Public opinion and 'domestic behaviour' had been subject to 'profound' change during the course of the war. Birth control had become a common rather than an 'exceptional characteristic of marital relations in nearly all sectors of society'.[83] Contraceptive literature and 'rubber shops' had become more prevalent, and sexual relations had become more casual. In 1918 the illegitimacy rate was 30 per cent higher than before the war. The divorce rate also increased by approximately 300 per cent between 1910 and 1920.[84] Churchmen were certainly not oblivious to the processes which had been set in motion and the challenges with which they were faced. We might note that the older generation of evangelical leaders was being replaced by 'a new generation of liberal evangelicals committed to ecumenism and a social application of the Gospel'.[85]

In a book entitled *Christian Ethics and Modern Problems*[86] W. R. Inge, the Dean of St Paul's and a well-known eugenicist, was quite explicit in identifying the First World War as an experience which had shaken not only the political but also the whole social structure. War had called into question prevailing values and traditions. This giant 'catastrophe' which had cast such a shadow on the 'old diplomacy' was also widely believed to have included the 'old religion'.[87] Christianity had failed to prevent the imperial powers from entering into a 'mutual suicide club' and clerics had usually fanned the patriotic flames. Christian ethics had been exposed to unprecedented scepticism and overt criticism. In part it was conceded that these developments had accelerated opinion which had been present for some time, but, over and above this, there had been 'a real emancipation from traditions which no longer corresponded with the new scientific knowledge, and with the new aspirations of a revolutionary epoch'.[88] A questioning, sceptical attitude seemed to have replaced the immutable authority of the pulpit. According to Inge, New Testament morality would have to 'stand its trial before the conscience of our generation, to be accepted or rejected on its merits as guide for the men and women of to-day'.[89] Among those issues of practical ethics with which Inge felt it necessary to engage was suicide and the 'closely connected' question of 'so-called euthanasia'. In his view this was an issue which Christianity had 'condemned' with 'particular severity'.[90] Many of the arguments against this practice were considered to have weakened considerably. The notion that an individual's 'eternal destiny' depended upon their state of mind at the moment at which they resigned from life was no longer regarded as being sufficiently convincing. The belief that suicide precluded the opportunity for repentance and absolution and should therefore be recognised as an act of supreme danger, was also rejected.[91] He was unable to endorse the view that the prolongation of suffering was willed by God 'for the benefit of the soul'.

Inge also cited other objections of a more practical nature. Notably, the perversity of the English law, whereby a man was liable to prosecution if he failed to put a suffering animal 'out of its misery', but was likely to be hanged if he took a similar course of action in the case of a terminally-ill cancer patient. These arguments provide a common theme in the British euthanasia debate. But like a number of those before him, Inge juxtaposed this form of individualistic and humanitarian euthanasia with arguments based on a cost benefit analysis of an individual's contribution to societal welfare. It was Inge's citation of Aristotle and Hume that seems to be of most significance with regard to the euthanasia debate of this period. The Aristotelian view that man had no right to deprive the state of his services was qualified with a passing reference to David Hume. One assumes Inge was alluding here to Hume's suggestion that suicide, in the case of an individual whose life was burdensome and no longer capable of promoting the interests of society, would enhance societal welfare rather than impoverish it.

We have seen that in the economic vicissitudes of Britain between the wars particular individuals were prepared to contemplate the non-voluntary mercy-killing of mental defectives. In part this might be seen as a radicalisation of the eugenic ideas which received a new impetus at this time, but there were other important considerations. For individuals such as A. F. Tredgold and R. J. A. Berry, who were prominent figures within the field of mental health, it seems likely that the lives of the profound mental defective were regarded as being genuinely pitiable, consequently an early death was to be regarded as merciful. But in the case of F. A. W. Gisborne, the proposal seems to have been predicated on a more utilitarian calculus. By killing defectives a financial burden to the nation would be relieved and so would a personal burden to the families who had to care for these individuals. Such proposals were clearly not endorsed widely.

Mercy-killing was not seen as a desirable or effective policy by the Eugenics Society; it was concerned with the most pronounced cases who were not regarded as the most dangerous from a eugenic perspective. It was considered highly unlikely that these individuals would ever reproduce. However, in the following years, proposals for non-voluntary euthanasia would persist and it is important therefore to have identified the complex rationale which underpinned these proposals. It has also been instructive to note that during this period, proposals for voluntary euthanasia tended to be distilled from those for non-voluntary euthanasia, rather than vice versa. Significantly, we see that even when individuals such as Gisborne and Inge advocated voluntary euthanasia, in addition to the relief of the individual's suffering, euthanasia was seen partly as an altruistic act which would be of benefit to others. Such sentiment was a continuation of the arguments raised in the course of the euthanasia debate of the 1870s; it has remained a persistent theme in the history of the British euthanasia movement.

Notes

1 See, for example, Ezekiel J. Emanuel, 'The history of euthanasia debates in the United States and Britain', *Annals of Internal Medicine*, 15 Nov. 1994, Vol. 121. No. 10, pp. 793–802; I. Van Der Sluis, 'The movement for euthanasia 1875–1975', *Janus*, 66, pp. 131–72.

2 Lionel Tollemache, 'The Cure for Incurables', *Fortnightly Review*, Feb. 1873, p. 219.

3 Charles Sorley, *The Letters of Charles Sorley* (Cambridge, 1919) p. 305.

4 On the role of political economy in military medicine see Roger Cooter, 'War and modern medicine', in W. F. Bynum and Roy Porter (eds), *Companion Encyclopedia of the History of Medicine* (London, 1993).

5 The epidemic was responsible for some 150,000 deaths in England and Wales.

6 See for example: 'Euthanasia', *BMJ*, 30 Nov. 1929, p. 1027; 'The right to die', *BMJ*, 4 Nov. 1911, pp. 1215–17.

7 One exception to this general rule was a letter to *The Lancet* in which the classical meaning was retained: 'Cocaine for euthanasia', *The Lancet*, 20 Sept. 1924, p. 629.

8 'The right to die', *BMJ*, 4 Nov. 1911, pp. 1215–17.

9 G. R. Searle, 'Eugenics and politics in the 1930s', *Annals of Science*, Vol. 36, 1979, pp. 159–69.

10 For a discussion of contemporaneous mercy-killing proposals for the mentally defective in a German context, see Michael Burleigh, *Death and Deliverance: Euthanasia in Germany 1900–45* (Cambridge, 1994) pp. 11–42.

11 John Stevenson, *British Society 1914–45* (London, [1984], 1990) p. 94.

12 *Ibid.*

13 'Eugenics and the war', *Eugenics Review*, Vol. 6, No. 3, Oct. 1914, p. 196.

14 Stevenson, *British Society*, p. 95.

15 *Eugenics Review*, Vol. 6, No. 3, Oct. 1914, p. 197.

16 *Ibid.*

17 Cited in Richard Soloway, *Demography and Degeneration* (Chapel Hill, 1990) p. 142.

18 *Ibid.*, p. 141.

19 *Eugenics Review*, Vol. 7, No. 2, 1915, p. 92.

20 Stevenson, *British Society*, p. 21.

21 C. W. Saleeby, 'The dysgenics of war', *Contemporary Review*, Vol. 107, 1915, p. 333.

22 John Keay, 'War and the burden of insanity', *The Journal of Mental Science*, Oct 1918, Vol. 64, No. 267, pp. 325–45.

23 *Ibid.*, p. 326.

24 *Ibid.*, p. 332.

25 *Ibid.*

26 See John Macnicol, 'Eugenics and the campaign for voluntary sterilisation in Britain between the wars', *Social History of Medicine*, Vol. 2, No. 2, (August, 1989) pp. 147–70.

27 For a discussion of the origins of the terms of mental deficiency see Mark Jackson, *The Borderland of Imbecility: Medicine, Society and the Fabrication of the Feeble-mind in Later Victorian and Edwardian England* (Manchester, 2000).

28 A. F. Tredgold, *Mental Deficiency: Amentia*, 4th edn (London, 1922) p. 93.

29 R. J. A. Berry, *Brain and Mind or the Nervous System of Man* (London, 1928) p. 524.

30 Tredgold, *Mental Deficiency*, 4th edn (London, 1922) pp. 94–5.

31 *Ibid.*, pp. 95–6.

32 Leonard Darwin, *The Need For Eugenic Reform* (London, 1926).

33 *Ibid.*, pp. 171–2.

34 The 1947 edition of Mental Deficiency, indicates that Tredgold had reversed his previous views and in fact advocated euthanasia for low-grade defectives. This is discussed in Chapter 5.

35 Tredgold, *Mental Deficiency*, p. 533.

36 See, 'Eugenics and the war', *Eugenics Review* Vol. 6, No. 3, Oct. 1914, pp. 197–8.

37 See, *Fourth Report of the Board of Control for the Year 1917* (London, 1918) pp. 14–25.

38 See, *Fifth Report of the Board of Control for the Year 1918* (London, 1919) p. 20.

39 *Ibid.*, p. 23.

40 *Ibid.*, p. 24.

41 *Ibid.*

42 *Ibid.*

43 *Ibid.*, p. 25.

44 *Ibid.*

45 *Ibid.*

46 F. A. W. Gisborne, *Democracy on Trial* (London, 1928).

47 *Ibid.*, p. v.

48 *Ibid.*, p. 210.

49 *Ibid.*, pp. 216–17.

50 *Ibid.*, pp. 219–20.

51 *Ibid.*, p. 220.

52 *Ibid.*, pp. 221–2.

53 *Ibid.*, p. 222.

54 Mathew Thomson, *The Problem of Mental Deficiency: Eugenics, Democracy, and Social Policy in Britain, c. 1870–1959* (Oxford, 1998).

55 The Committee was under the chairmanship of Sir Arthur Wood.

56 See Macnicol, 'Eugenics', p. 160.

57 1929 *Joint Committee Report on Mental Deficiency* (3 vols. HMSO) p. 81.

58 *Ibid.*, p. 75.

59 *Ibid.*, p. 83.

60 Macnicol, 'Eugenics', p. 154.

61 See Greta Jones, *Social Hygiene in Twentieth-Century Britain* (London, 1986) p. 85.

62 *Joint Committee Report*, p. 82.

63 R. J. A. Berry obituaries, *BMJ*, 6 Oct 1962, pp. 930–1; *The Lancet*, 13 Oct. 1962, p. 789.

64 See Berry, *Brain and Mind*, pp. 513–23.

65 *Eugenics Review*, 1930, p. 6

66 For discussion of Ewald Meltzer's *The Problem of Curtailment of Life Unworthy*

of Life, see Michael Burleigh, *Death and Deliverance: 'Euthanasia' in Germany c. 1900–1945* (Cambridge, 1994) pp. 21–5.

67 Binding was a lawyer and former President of the Reichsgericht; Hoche was Professor of Psychiatry at Freiburg University.

68 Karl Binding and Alfred Hoche, *Permission for the Destruction of Worthless Life, its Extent and Form* (Leipzig, 1920), cited in J. Noakes and G. Pridham (eds), *Nazism 1919–1945, Vol. 3, Foreign Policy, War and Racial Extermination: A Documentary Reader* (Exeter, 1988, reprinted 1991) pp. 996–8.

69 Cited in Burleigh, *Death and Deliverance*, p. 17.

70 *Ibid.*

71 Cited in Noakes and Pridham, *Nazism* Vol. 3, p. 1000.

72 Gisborne, *Democracy on Trial*, p. 210.

73 *Ibid.*, p. 218.

74 *Ibid.*, p. 213.

75 *Ibid.*, pp. 213–14.

76 *Ibid.*, p. 214.

77 *Ibid.*, p. 182.

78 Alan Wilkinson, *The Church of England and the First World War* (London [1978], 1996) p. 173.

79 Pat Jalland, *Death in the Victorian Family* (Oxford, 1996) p. 380.

80 Cited in Wilkinson, *The Church of England*, p. 183.

81 John Stevenson, *British Society*, p. 356.

82 Stuart Mews, 'Religious life between the wars, 1920–1940', in Sheridan Gilley and W. J. Sheils (eds), *A History of Religion in Britain* (Oxford, 1994) p. 449.

83 Richard Soloway, *Demography and Degeneration*, p. 193.

84 Wilkinson, *The Church of England*, p. 105.

85 *Ibid.*, p. 7.

86 W. R. Inge, *Christian Ethics and Modern Problems* (London, 1930).

87 *Ibid.*, preface.

88 *Ibid.*

89 *Ibid.*

90 *Ibid.*, p. 372.

91 *Ibid.*, pp. 372–3.

4

The attempt to legalise voluntary euthanasia, 1931–36

For over sixty years the Voluntary Euthanasia Legalisation Society has provided an institutional forum within which discussions on euthanasia have taken place in Great Britain.[1] Although the Society was not founded until 1935, the germ of the movement can be located in the 1931 Presidential address of Dr Charles Killick Millard to the Annual General Meeting of the Society of Medical Officers of Health.[2] This address in which Millard advocated the 'Legalisation of Voluntary Euthanasia' provoked the first sustained, nationwide euthanasia debate. The debate occupied substantial column-inches in all the leading medical journals, daily newspapers and popular periodicals, eliciting a broad spectrum of opinion from among the medical profession, ecclesiastics and lay persons. Within four years of his address Millard and a small clique of colleagues drawn from the intellectual circles of Leicester were mooting the formation of a Euthanasia Society. In October 1935, following the offer of substantial financial assistance from a terminally-ill London gentleman,[3] the Voluntary Euthanasia Legalisation Society was formally established.

From its inception the Society professed a desire to attract a large membership which would demonstrate 'the strength of public support behind the movement'.[4] It would be misleading, however, to suggest that the Society was a truly grass-roots, populist movement. During the 1930s it conspicuously refrained from demonstrations of popular support and abstained from the use of vigorous advertising campaigns among the general populace. The Society's chosen tactic was to secure legislative reform by establishing a network of distinguished sympathisers able to influence policy at high levels, rather than by means of populist pressure from below. Consequently, although there was a far from negligible cate-

gory of 'ordinary' members, it seems prudent to focus prosopographical analysis on the Executive Committee, the Consultative
Medical Council, the Vice-Presidents, and the Literary Group,
which appear to have constituted the active membership of the
Society. We should note, however, that even within these four categories, there were definite gradations of significance among the
membership. A small number of individuals were heavily engaged
with the Society's work, while a considerable number of others were
remarkably passive, appearing to do little except consent to the use
of their name in Societal literature.

At the core of the Executive Committee were the Honorary
Secretary, Dr Charles Killick Millard, Medical Officer of Health for
Leicester 1901–35, and the Chairman, Mr C. J. Bond, Consulting
Surgeon to the Leicester Royal Infirmary. Both of these men were
distinguished medical personalities, well-known in public health
circles for their reformist attitudes and outspoken positions on a
number of medico-social issues.

Throughout his career, Millard held numerous positions within
his locality. He had served as President of the Leicester Literary and
Philosophical Society, Leicester Rotary Club, the Leicester
Temperance Society, the Leicester Band of Hope Union, the
Leicester Medical Society, Chairman of the Leicester and Rutland
Division of the British Medical Association, and Vice-President of
the Public Health Section in 1922 and 1932.[5] It was during his time
as Medical Officer of Health for Leicester, however, that Millard had
earned himself a nationwide reputation as something of a maverick,
opposing the policy of compulsory smallpox vaccination, on sophisticated, though controversial epidemiological grounds.[6] He had also
helped pioneer experimental farm colonies for consumptives as a
method of treating tuberculosis.[7] Further indications of his diverse
interests and reforming credentials are provided by his efforts to
promote the consumption of horseflesh as a substitute for other
varieties of meat during the period of wartime shortages,[8] and his
advocacy of prohibition.[9]

It was on the question of birthcontrol, however, that Millard
had been perhaps most outspoken. His concern with the issue had
become manifest in the period immediately following the First
World War. As noted in the previous chapter, this was a time at
which ethical reappraisal seemed particularly propitious. To Millard
it seemed as though a 'new era' was 'dawning, prejudice and obscu-

rantism' were 'giving way, and the light of civilisation and common sense' was 'at last breaking through'.[10] He considered it an 'inherent and inalienable right' of all married couples to decide when it was advisable to 'exercise the privilege of having children'. Indeed, because it required 'intelligence, forethought and self-control' Millard believed that birth control was indicative of 'an altogether higher morality than the old fashioned practice of reckless and uncontrolled breeding'.[11] The issue was also intimately related to questions of poverty, and child and maternal welfare, which tended to be adversely affected by excessive fertility amongst the lower classes.[12] In addition, there was a strong eugenic dimension to his advocacy of birth control. On numerous occasions, he suggested that it was 'quality and not quantity of the human species' which the world required.[13] He had made clear his view that the possibility of increasing fertility among the eugenically desirable was unlikely. There was no evidence to suggest that the inverse relationship between quality and quantity was likely to change. Only by advocating the use of birth control among the 'less efficient classes' could the Eugenics Society really hope to make a difference.[14] In fact, Richard Soloway's comprehensive study of the inter-relationships between the birth control and eugenics movements,[15] has identified Millard as one of the principal figures responsible for manoeuvring the Eugenics Society into the advocacy of birth control following the First World War. Millard's advocacy of eugenic policies also extended to support for the sterilisation of the feeble-minded.[16]

Mr C. J. Bond, had enjoyed a similarly distinguished career. He was twice President of the Leicester Literary and Philosophical Society, Vice-President of several temperance societies, President of the Society for the Study of Inebriety, Fellow of University College London, life member of the British Association for the Advancement of Science, Vice-Chairman to the Ministry of Health's medical Consultative Council, and for eight years he served on the Medical Research Council of the Privy Council. He was also Deputy Chairman of the Industrial Research Board, member of the Departmental Commission on the Cause and Prevention of Blindness, the Departmental Committee on Cancer, and was a Vice-President of the Eugenics Society. If these posts had not kept him busy enough, between 1878 and 1939, he managed to write 'no less than 157 essays and memoirs' which 'ranged over the whole subject of health, national as well as individual'.[17] A seemingly earnest man, Bond's recreational activities were recorded in *Who's Who* as 'Sociology, and research in heredity and other scientific subjects'. Like Millard, he was a prominent advocate of birth control, serving on the National Birth Control Council, and had also been a central figure in steering the Eugenics Society towards the adoption of a pro-contraception platform. A vehement advocate of eugenic sterilisation,[18] Bond had allegedly persuaded a group of blind men to undergo the operation.[19] He believed that 'man was being called upon to play an increasing part in the control of human evolution and human destiny; and that among the duties and responsibilities which he [would] be called upon to undertake, those concerned with entrance into and exit from life [would] be some of the most important'.[20] This quotation provides an indication of the way in which several advocates of euthanasia were inclined to see physician assisted suicide as one element of a broader medico-social endeavour. For most of the 1930s, this duo of Millard and Bond constituted the driving force of the euthanasia movement.

The other members of the Executive Committee appear to have been associates of Millard and Bond, drawn from Leicester's tight network of intellectuals. Astley V. Clarke was an Honorary Physician at the Leicester Royal Infirmary, and had served as President of the Leicester Literary and Philosophical Society (1912), President of the Leicester Medical Society (1911), and Deputy Chairman of the Leicester City Health Committee.[21] He had also been Vice-President and Chairman of the Council of University College Leicester. One assumes that this would have brought him into contact with Revd Dr R. F. Rattray, another Executive Committee member, who between 1921 and 1931 was the first Principal of University College, Leicester.[22] Prior to this Rattray had been Minister at the Unitarian Chapel of Great Meeting, where Millard had been a regular worshipper and Chairman of the Vestry. Two other ecclesiastics served on the Committee: Canon F. R. C. Payne, Canon Chancellor of Leicester Cathedral between 1931 and 1954; and the Revd A. S. Hurn. Rattray's successor as Principal at University College, Leicester was Frederick Attenborough, who was also a member of the Society's Executive Committee; and the remaining member was the Honorary Solicitor, H. T. Cooper, about whom biographical details are unfortunately elusive.

With the exception of C. E. Goddard's brief flirtation with the subject, euthanasia, in the mercy-killing sense, had failed to engage the medical profession with any vigour. Yet during the 1930s the impetus for the legalisation of voluntary euthanasia came firmly from within this hitherto disinterested profession. Clearly there was a strong medical component to the Executive Committee, and alongside this was the Consultative Medical Council. Exactly why so many prominent figures should have felt inclined to engage with this issue is extremely difficult to determine, and no doubt there were many different motives. Nevertheless, it is clear that all members of the Council were distinguished figures, with numerous fellows of the Royal College of Physicians, Surgeons and of the Royal Society. A high proportion were also active in the field of public health. This leads one to ask whether the euthanasia movement should be seen as part of the 'social hygiene' movement of the early twentieth century to which Greta Jones has drawn attention.[23]

According to Jones, this movement fused the environmentalist

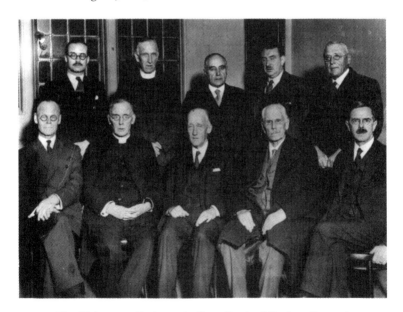

1   The Voluntary Euthanasia (Legalisation) Society Executive Committee. Back row, L–R: Lord Listowel, Canon F. R. C. Payne, H. T. Cooper, A. Percy Groves, Dr Astley V. Clarke. Front row, L–R: Dr C. Killick Millard, Canon Peter Green, Lord Ponsonby, C. J. Bond, Revd Dr A. S. Hurn

concerns of the 'public health and sanitary reform movement' of the late nineteenth century with the hereditarian ideas of the late nineteenth and early twentieth centuries. Such a paradigm is initially rather appealing bearing in mind the backgrounds of Millard and Bond. In fact there was considerable overlap between the membership of the Voluntary Euthanasia Legalisation Society and the Eugenics Society. A conservative estimate would suggest that at least 12 per cent of the Voluntary Euthanasia Legalisation Society were also members of the Eugenics Society. Amongst the Society's Vice-Presidents, we can also identify figures such as Sir W. Arbuthnot Lane, President of the New Health Society; an organisation which Jones sees as central to the social hygiene movement. Despite the shared personnel, Jones's depiction of a social hygiene movement has not gone unchallenged. Historians have suggested that the term is as confusing as it is revealing,[24] tending to gloss over the complexities of what were in fact very broad churches. This chapter argues that although relationships between the euthanasia and eugenics movements did exist, they were complex. We must also recognise that while numerous public health officials can be found among the ranks of the Society, the majority of the profession chose not to join. The membership of experts from the diverse fields of nervous diseases, obstetrics, gynaecology, epidemiology and vital statistics, surgery, physiology, ophthalmology, and general practice, would also seem to question the inclusion of euthanasia in a social hygiene paradigm.

In addition to the Society's medical component, there was a literary group which included about a dozen well-known authors. Again it is not immediately apparent why such individuals should have felt inclined to join the Society. But, it is clear that among this group, there were a number of progressive reformers such as Vera Brittain, Henry Havelock Ellis, Cicely Hamilton, Laurence Housman, and H. G. Wells. This cluster of feminists, pacifists, eugenists, Fabians, and advocates of birth control would seem to indicate that the Voluntary Euthanasia Legalisation Society was seen as a rather progressive movement. We should note, however, that as was the case with the Society's Consultative Medical Council and Vice-Presidents, many members of this group had been approached by members of the Executive Committee and personally invited to join. They were selected primarily on the basis of their eminence in their own particular field, as opposed to a field which was necessarily pertinent to euthanasia. The Society believed that such a diverse membership would illustrate the widespread support which the Society enjoyed among a plethora of distinguished figures in a multitude of different walks of life. They were identified as potential members following the perusal of *Who's Who* by members of the Executive Committee. Frequently these members were entirely inactive, although there were notable exceptions such as Havelock Ellis who produced several articles on the subject.

The progressive qualities of the literary group were also shared by the Society's list of Vice-Presidents which included such figures as Miss Eleanor Rathbone MP, George Bernard Shaw and Professor G. M. Trevelyan. Despite this, the Vice-Presidents were a very diverse collection of individuals of all political hues, ranging from left-wing intellectuals such as Professor Harold Laski, to the future Conservative peer, Lord Woolton of Liverpool. Indeed the Society's Vice-Presidents included no less than ten peers. Although one cannot be sure, it is likely that their membership had been influenced by Lord Moynihan, who as a past President of the Royal College of Surgeons had been invited to be the first President of the Voluntary Euthanasia Legalisation Society and accepted.

The function of the Society was to promote a Parliamentary Bill which would legalise voluntary euthanasia for fully *compos mentis* adult patients suffering from an incurable and fatal illness characterised by severe pain. The Voluntary Euthanasia (Legalisation) Bill was introduced to the House of Lords in 1936, and following a lively debate on its second reading, on 1 December 1936, was defeated by thirty-five votes to fourteen.

This chapter sets out to map the nature of the discourse on euthanasia, up to and including the House of Lords debate. In distinction to the discussions of the immediate post-war years, the debate of the nineteen-thirties was concerned primarily with voluntary euthanasia for terminally-ill patients, rather than with non-voluntary euthanasia for the mentally defective. Although this was a period during which the eugenics movement was enjoying something of a resurgence,[25] the principal catalyst for this debate seems to have been an acute awareness of epidemiological patterns. To be more explicit, persistent increases in the number of deaths from cancer, a 'notoriously painful disease', were identified as fuelling the need for euthanasia. Of course epidemiological shifts alone cannot explain why significant numbers of prominent medical figures were increasingly sympathetic to a proposal which clearly constituted a profound alteration to the profession's ethical code; a code which had persistently placed the wilful curtailment of life outside the physician's remit. But, as the previous chapter indicated, the experience of unprecedented human loss during the First World War, combined with accompanying secular trends, had seemed to usher in a wave of ethical reappraisal opening the way for the discussion of a host of medico-social issues. This was in fact an interpretation which Millard endorsed repeatedly.

> That gigantic cataclysm, the Great War, undoubtedly had a loosening and disintegrating effect upon old-established ideas, such as we have never seen before. The change in public opinion since the war, in connection with the subject of birth control, is an illustration of this. In some respects, birth control raised similar issues, as regards orthodox 'morality', as does voluntary euthanasia.[26]

During this period, doctors seem to have become more sympathetic to active euthanasia, which for the first time became a practical proposal. But, in spite of all the enthusiasm and support which was generated, there remained strong opposition from within the profession. While there was no concerted anti-euthanasia movement at this time, considerable debate took place and was recorded in the pages of the medical press, which this chapter will outline in some detail. Medical objection was indeed strong, and the defeat of the Voluntary Euthanasia (Legalisation) Bill defeat is usually attributed to the speeches made against the motion by two eminent medical peers:[27] Lord Dawson, a former President of the Royal College of Physicians, and Lord Horder, the outstanding clinician of his time and one of the most well-known figures in medicine. These speeches, which eloquently summarised the medical and practical objections to euthanasia certainly carried considerable weight, but it is suggested here that the reasons for the Bill's defeat are more complex.

A persistent theme of the modern euthanasia debate has been the clash between the advocates of physician-assisted suicide, motivated by humanitarian concern, and religious opponents who have repeatedly condemned the deliberate precipitation of death. Most resolute among this latter group has been the Catholic Church which has provided stout opposition to the attempts to legalise mercy-killing and a number of other medico-social issues, becoming particularly vocal following the 1929 Papal Bull against eugenics.

Opposition of this nature peppered the euthanasia debate of the 1930s and was particularly apparent in publications such as *The Universe* and the *Catholic Medical Journal*.

Among the Protestant Churches, however, there appears to have been much sympathy towards the euthanasia movement. As we have already noted, there were three clergymen serving on the Executive Committee of the Society, and among the increasing number of liberal theologians who had risen to prominence since the First World War, there was considerable support. Although there was a strong religious component to the euthanasia debate, the Voluntary Euthanasia Legalisation Society was comparatively successful in combating theological opposition. This is certainly not to suggest that there was anything resembling a sympathetic consensus among the Protestant Churches, but it should be noted that theological issues did not feature prominently in the Lords' debate. Nevertheless, the arguments which Society members employed as a mechanism for circumventing the sanctity of human life issue, tended, not infrequently, to expose them to a number of other objections.

A notable feature of the euthanasia debate from the 1870s onwards, which enjoyed a great deal of currency during the 1930s, was the citation of eminent historical figures extolling the virtues of self-murder in particular circumstances. Such historical references purported to demonstrate that euthanasia had not always been subject to moral censure, indeed it had been positively lauded by several great thinkers. One can appreciate the *ad hominem* appeal of such rhetoric, but the examples cited were often replete with altruistic sentiments which suggested that self-murder was a duty when life had become excessively burdensome to family, friends and society. Notions of this variety surfaced during the Lords debate and raised the eyebrows of the opponents of euthanasia who were concerned about the normative dimension of euthanasia.

One stage beyond this, was the so-called slippery-slope argument. This suggested that once voluntary euthanasia for the *compos mentis* had been legalised, there would be a move towards the legalisation of non-voluntary euthanasia for defectives. In order to avoid any confusion it is important to make a distinction between two varieties of slippery-slope argument. The first suggests that there is a logical connection between the two practices outlined above; once the first is legalised, the second will inevitably follow. Although particular arguments used to justify voluntary euthanasia may be transferred to the case of non-voluntary euthanasia for the *non compos mentis*, the logical slippery slope is an argument which is very difficult to sustain. The second form of slippery slope, and the one which is pertinent to this chapter, is a descriptive one. It suggests, merely, that particular advocates of the legalisation of voluntary euthanasia saw this as a first step to be followed by the legalisation of non-voluntary euthanasia for the mentally and physically defective. In part the notion of a slippery slope had been fostered by Catholic opponents who were keen to depict euthanasia, birth control and sterilisation as a concerted assault upon Divine Providence. There were, however, more substantive reasons for its prevalence. With a degree of regularity, prominent figures within the euthanasia movement tended to reveal the inflationary potential of a Bill which was in the first instance concerned solely and incontrovertibly with voluntary mercy-killing for the terminally ill.

Usually those advocating non-voluntary euthanasia for defectives did so on humanitarian grounds. They suggested that by giving euthanasia to grossly deformed and defective infants, the recipients would be spared much suffering. The mere fact that the *non compos mentis* were unable to express a desire to die, was considered insufficient reason to preclude such individuals from the relief available to the *compos mentis*; a third party would simply be required to act in their best interest. But, in a similar fashion to the euthanasia debates of preceding eras, it was not uncommon for the interests of family, friends and society to be included in the calculus which would decide whether non-voluntary euthanasia could be justified in individual cases. Eugenic concerns also surfaced, but as we have seen from the above, it is misleading to label all proposals for the non-voluntary mercy-killing of defectives as eugenic euthanasia. The primary objective was usually not an aggregate improvement of the race. However, a desire to reduce the overall number of defectives in society did feature in the rhetoric of some advocates. Euthanasia and eugenics certainly enjoyed a relationship of sorts during the 1930s, but it must be treated carefully. This chapter suggests that objections to the altruistic dimension of euthanasia and the fear of a slippery slope provided considerable grounds for opposing to the Voluntary Euthanasia (Legalisation) Bill of 1936 and did more to defeat it than has hitherto been recognised.

The proposal outlined by Charles Killick Millard in his Presidential Address of 1931 was simply that fully *compos mentis* adult patients suffering from an incurable and terminal illness 'which usually entails a slow and painful death, should be allowed by law ... to substitute for the slow and painful death a quick and painless one'. The proposed Bill stipulated that the patient desiring euthanasia would be required to sign a request form in the presence of two witnesses, which would be sent along with medical certificates to a referee appointed by the Ministry of Health who would either issue or deny a licence for euthanasia. The decision would be entirely voluntary. This was deemed to be not only an 'act of mercy', but 'a matter of elementary human right'.[28] The urgency of this measure was alleged to be underpinned by observable epidemiological trends. An increase in the incidence of cancer in recent years was identified as the principal cause for a rise in the proportion of painful deaths. Statistics from the Registrar General's Office illustrated that the number of deaths from malignant disease in England and Wales in 1929 (the last year for which statistics were available) was 'higher than ever before', at some 56,896. Of those deaths occurring over the age of forty, one out of every seven was the result of cancer.[29] Much of the 'sting' of death lay in this protracted suffering which preceded the final passing of the patient. Citing C. E. Goddard's paper of 1901, which had drawn attention to the incidence of malignant disease as an argument in favour of mercy-killing, Millard noted that far from matters having improved in the intervening thirty years, the number of people dying from cancer in proportion to population size was 'almost twice as great as it was at the time when Dr Goddard wrote'.[30]

That attention should be drawn to these epidemiological trends was perhaps not surprising bearing in mind the involvement of several Society members with the Ministry of Health's Cancer Committee. C. J. Bond, Sir George Buchanan, and Professor Major Greenwood (Professor of Epidemiology and Vital Statistics, University College London) had all been members of the Committee, and Millard and R. Veitch Clark (MOH for Manchester) both served on the Medical Officers of Health's Sub-Committee which was chaired by Buchanan.[31] The members of this sub-committee had contributed to the work of the central committee by initiating investigations and collecting data from their own localities. As we have noted, the Voluntary Euthanasia Legalisation

Society was very much a Leicester-based organisation in its early years. Leicester happened to be a city in which 'special' cancer clinics had been established and where efforts had been made to educate the public about cancer, with notices and leaflets describing the symptoms of cancer and the objects of the clinic being sent to factories.[32] Indeed, it would seem that among the medical members of the Society, there was a fair degree of familiarity with the disease.

The number of deaths attributable to cancer had certainly increased, but the age-structure of Great Britain had also changed significantly. A higher proportion of old people ensured that there was greater susceptibility to the disease. Thus, when mortality statistics were standardised to take these changes into account, the sharp increase which the crude death rates revealed was moderated substantially. Improvements in pathological knowledge and technical equipment, combined with the 'newer bases of classification and improvements in diagnosis' meant that it was extremely difficult to determine precise epidemiological patterns. The Chief Medical Officer's Annual Report, had suggested that the 'more cautious ask: "Is cancer increasing?" The less cautious declare that "Cancer is increasing by leaps and bounds."'[33] Millard was evidently among the latter category. But, at a certain level, the question of whether or not the virulence of cancer had increased was rather unimportant. The fact that more people were suffering from cancer, irrespective of changes in age distribution, ensured that as far as Millard was concerned, there was a concomitant increase in the proportion of painful deaths, leading him to the conclusion that the appropriate moment had arrived at which to discuss the legalisation of voluntary euthanasia.

The proposal to legalise voluntary euthanasia clearly did not sit comfortably alongside the Hippocratic Oath. Yet it was unusual for supporters of euthanasia to propose the outright rejection of the Oath. Lord Moynihan, a past President of the Royal College of Surgeons, and first President of the Voluntary Euthanasia Legalisation Society, had chosen to ignore the issue by claiming, rather dubiously, that the proposed reform was not a fundamental one.[34] A more common approach, however, was to bypass the Hippocratic Oath by appealing to the doctrine of double effect. This was a technique which had been used by the supporters of euthanasia from the time of S. D. Williams onwards. It suggested that while the physician could administer analgesics in order to relieve pain,

Table 1 Recorded deaths per million from cancer in England and Wales, 1847–1927[34]

1847–50	274	1906–10	939
1851–55	306	1911–15*	1,055
1856–60	327	1916–20*	1,182
1861–65	367	1921–25	1,269
1866–70	403	1921	1,215
1871–75	445	1922	1,229
1876–80	494	1923	1,267
1881–85	548	1924	1,297
1886–90	632	1925	1,336
1891–95	712	1926	1,362
1896–00	800	1927	1,376
1901–05	867		

*The mortality for the years 1915–1920 relates to civilians only.
Source: Chief Medical Officer's Annual Report 1927, p. 99.

Table 2 Annual mortality from cancer per million living 1925-30, crude and standardised rates

Year	Crude	Standardised
1925	1,336	1,002
1926	1,363 (26)	999 (–3)
1927	1,376 (14)	996 (–3)
1928	1,425 (49)	1,011 (15)
1929	1,437 (12)	1,010 (–1)
1930	1,454 (17)	1,003 (–7)

Source: Abridged table from *Chief Medical Officer's Annual Report 1935* (London, 1936).

tolerance to narcotics, particularly morphia tended to be established very rapidly, requiring successively larger doses in order to relieve pain, until perilously large doses would be required in order to achieve any palliation. According to Millard, a 'merciful doctor is in a grave dilemma. He may be said to be hovering on the brink of manslaughter.'[35] C. J. Bond concurred on this issue, claiming that the ethical distinction between pain relief and accelerating death was not clearly defined.[36] Such arguments were not without validity, but they could not disguise the fact that the goal of the Voluntary Euthanasia Legalisation Society was not merely to ensure that physicians, who inadvertently brought about the premature death of a terminally-ill patient while attempting to ease their suffering, were protected from prosecution.

Of course one may engage in protracted philosophical debate about whether there is a meaningful distinction between the intended and unintended consequences of a physician's actions in such cases,[37] but the fact remains that the Voluntary Euthanasia Legalisation Society was advocating the deliberate and wilful precipitation of death. That a few hours or even days of a patient's life might be lost as a consequence of palliative care was deemed justifiable by all but the most resolute opponents of interference with Divine Providence. Lord Dawson during the course of his forceful speech against the Voluntary Euthanasia (Legalisation) Bill was explicit on the acceptability of a physician's actions in these circumstances, noting that the 'present age' was a 'courageous one' with a 'different sense of values' from the ages which had gone before. 'It looks upon life more from the point of view of quality than quantity.' We might also note that despite Millard's protestations, one is hardly overwhelmed by the number of manslaughter prosecutions against physicians who had accidentally shortened the lives of their terminally-ill patients.

Perhaps not surprisingly, the British Medical Association was unwilling to endorse the objectives of the euthanasia movement, but it was prepared to oversee an active debate of this issue, and provided the Voluntary Euthanasia Legalisation Society with a room at BMA House, free of charge, in which to hold its first public meeting. Much of the ensuing medical discussion took place in this sort of arena and was reported in the medical press, usually without comment.

At a meeting of the Hunterian Society on 16 November 1936 the motion 'That the practice of voluntary euthanasia would be unjustifiable' was debated and received considerable support on medical and practical grounds. The reform proposed by the Voluntary Euthanasia Legalisation Society had stipulated that the patient desiring euthanasia should be experiencing pain, but it was extremely difficult to ascertain when this reached intolerable proportions. Nor was it clear whether the patient or the physician should be the ultimate arbiter on this matter. Such an objection was perhaps rather pedantic, as the Bill also stipulated that the illness must be of a terminal nature, but this does touch upon another issue of considerable importance.

From reading the speeches and publications of the Voluntary Euthanasia Legalisation Society, one gains the impression that owing to the increased incidence of cancer, the frequency of agonising deaths had multiplied astronomically. While conceding that enormous strides had been made in 'preventive', 'curative' and palliative medicine, Millard remained convinced that 'vast numbers of human beings' were 'doomed to end their earthly existence by a lingering, painful and often agonising form of death'.[38] This view was not unanimously supported. During the Lords debate, Lord Dawson sought to clarify this issue. He suggested that the impression was often given that acute pain was a far more frequent characteristic of disease than was really the case. 'In relation to cancer especially, it would not be correct to say that most cases of cancer are characterised by agonising pain.'[39]

Even in those cases where acute pain was evident, the stark choice between an agonising death and euthanasia, which the Society had done so much to propagate, was considered inappropriate by several medical authorities. Both Lord Dawson and Lord Horder alluded to the improvements which had been made in palliative care, offering a middle course between the Manichaean options presented by Millard.

Another interesting response which seems to have aroused little interest, was advanced in a letter to the editor of *The Lancet*, which raised the possibility of surgical pain relief. It suggested that a bilateral chordotomy carried out below the 'fifth cervical segment of the spinal chord' would serve to alleviate the pain of any local disease situated below this level. This letter was not intended as an argument against the aims and objectives of the Voluntary Euthanasia Legalisation Society, but with regard to conditions such as 'inoperable carcinoma of the pelvic organs' the possibility of surgical pain relief did 'seem to limit the field of their concerns very considerably'.[40] The Society as a whole failed to address this issue, and one assumes that this was because successes in palliative care tended to detract from the case for voluntary euthanasia.

Concerns had also been raised that a patient suffering fits of melancholia might desire euthanasia during a spell of dark depression, but in a 'brighter period' might not contemplate such a step.[41]

This in fact neglected a number of the safeguards outlined in the proposed Bill. The patient desiring euthanasia would be required to make written application to a euthanasia referee. The referee would then conduct an interview with the patient, which one assumes would ascertain whether the applicant was of sound mind. Permission to receive euthanasia would not operate 'until the expiration of seven days from the date on which the referee sends the permit to the patient and the referee shall on sending the permit notify the nearest relative of the patient that permission has been granted'.[42] Such a protracted exercise would certainly provide the opportunity for a change of mind. Within three days of the receipt of such a notice, the patient's nearest relative was also able to apply to a court of summary jurisdiction, alleging that a particular condition had not been met, and under these circumstances the court might cancel the permit.

But even if the patient was absolutely rational and lucid, there was of course the possibility that a doctor might make an incorrect diagnosis. As Lord Horder suggested, the 'fatal character and incurability of disease is never more than an estimate based upon experience, and how fallacious experience may be in medicine only those who have had a great deal of experience fully realise'.[43] Doctors were certainly not infallible and lives might be sacrificed which might conceivably be saved. Millard conceded as much, but in all 'grave decisions' human error was a possibility, and the sufferer would have to take the risk. Doctors already faced such difficulties when deciding whether or not to undertake a major surgical operation 'fraught with danger to life'.[44]

To a certain extent this was true, but there was a qualitative difference between these two scenarios. In the case of a major surgical operation, the objective was to prolong life, in which case the risk could be justified upon prevailing ethical grounds, while in the case of euthanasia, the intention was to curtail life, which fell outside the doctor's remit.

Occasionally it was suggested that euthanasia might also weaken the impetus for research to develop new cures.[45] Such arguments were a little simplistic, as euthanasia and biomedical research were not necessarily mutually exclusive. It was quite plausible, however, that diseases which were currently incurable, might be curable in the future. Opponents pointed to the fact that in the past hundred years, unprecedented developments had been made in medical science.[46] But this was also a rather weak objection. The recipients of euthanasia would be those in the last throes of a painful and terminal illness. Such patients could not wait around for a cure. Their imminent death was incontrovertible and the dispute centred on the circumstances of that death. In the event of cures being developed, the law would become redundant and would fall into disuse and could also be repealed.

Despite the deflection of particular arguments, other objections proliferated, several of which seemed to carry considerable weight. Notable among these was the suggestion that the legalisation of euthanasia would deny terminally-ill patients all hope. 'It would introduce a very disturbing element in the household of the patient ... [and] the whole procedure would add very much to the patient's distress and to the doctor's difficulties.' This was, and remains, a powerful argument against euthanasia. Perhaps more surprisingly, objections were raised that the proposed reform did not go far enough, it left out 'many patients who were a burden both to themselves and others'.[47] This was certainly not a mainstream objection to the proposed legalisation of voluntary euthanasia, but it was an issue with considerable bearing, to which we shall return.

For Millard and a number of others, the treatment accorded to terminally-ill human beings was deplorable in comparison to the case of an animal which had been hopelessly injured, or which was suffering from an incurable and painful disease where 'common humanity demands that we should "put the poor creature out of its pain". This is not only regarded as an act of mercy, but as a positive duty, neglect of which amount to actual cruelty.'[48] Human beings on the other hand were forced to endure the intense pain, suffering and indignity associated with terminal illnesses. In the words of Sir W. Arbuthnot Lane, 'If you allowed a dog or cat to linger in pain, the SPCA would be down on you like a shot.' Precisely the same example was used by Lord Denman in the Lords' debate of December 1936, but despite its frequent employment it was an analogy that was open to question. Catholics in particular were keen to point to a theological distinction between the morality of killing animals and humans. Although an appealing argument, the animal analogy is tenable only if one assumes that man has no higher destiny than a 'brute beast'. It was consequently unable to make any significant impact upon received 'Christian Wisdom'. The *Catholic Medical Journal* was quite explicit on this issue: 'Man has dominion over the lower creatures and can, within the limits laid down by right reason, put them to death for his food, his clothing, or even for his sport, but no such right does man possess over his own life or the lives of others.'[49]

Ethical arguments constantly stuttered in the face of Christian opposition, but Millard was quite prepared to fight his corner, launching a strong assault upon alleged Christian hypocrisy concerning the sanctity of human life. He argued that if this was really a concept which did not admit of degrees, then the failure of the Church to condemn capital punishment was anomalous to say the least. The argument concerning the 'infringement' of the Divine prerogative was also considered to be rather suspect, and lacking in coherence while the Christian Church tolerated, 'and indeed sanctioned, the wholesale taking of human life under the guise of war'.[50]

Millard was the son of minister, and throughout his life a pious man, but he was unable to accept a number of the medieval theological arguments which Catholic opponents of euthanasia were inclined to advance. He rejected the argument of St Augustine that the Biblical injunction 'Thou shalt not kill' applied to suicide, arguing that there was a profound difference between murder and suicide. This lay in the fact that murder was an act committed against another individual which deprived him of the 'most precious thing in life', that is life itself. In the case of suicide, no other party was necessarily injured 'in any way', the life which was taken was one's own. It was 'noteworthy that in the Revised Version of Ex. 20.13, "Thou shalt not kill" is translated "Thou shalt do no murder"'.[51]

For those Catholics who were prepared to concede that there was distinction to be drawn between murder and suicide, this by no means excused the 'sinfulness' of the latter. A letter to the *Leicester Evening Mail*, which cited the *Summa Theologica* in which St Thomas Aquinas had given three reasons for the sinfulness of suicide, provides a striking example:

1. It is an act against the profoundest natural inclination, for self preservation is called the first law of nature, and also against the love of self which charity requires. Moreover, because charity to self is more obligatory than charity to the neighbour, suicide is a more serious sin than other forms of homicide.
2. It is an offence against the community, which has a right to be benefited by the lives of its members and to receive a return for the

protection and assistance it affords them. The suicide deprives his fellow man of an example of fortitude, or at least of the opportunity of showing charity and mercy to the needy.

3. It is a grave injury against the rights of God, for it usurps His authority, refuses Him the authority, refuses Him the service He desires, spurns the gift He has bestowed, dishonours the image of God (Gen. ix. 6), and destroys the property of God: 'Thou, O Lord, hast the power of life and death.' (Wisd. xxi. 13)[52]

For others, the Catholic stance seemed excessively inflexible and outdated. As Dr A. S. Hurn of Leicester suggested, moral judgements could not ultimately depend upon 'custom or prejudice', they should be related to 'the ever-advancing enlightenment of the conscience of mankind.'[53] Nor was the Revd Dr R. F. Rattray able to identify any moral or religious objection, and found it unthinkable that a Beneficent Providence 'wills that the physical sufferings of humanity in the process of dying should unnecessarily be prolonged'.[54] To bolster this circumvention of Christian opposition, the Voluntary Euthanasia Legalisation Society published a statement on the ethical aspect of euthanasia signed by fifteen prominent religious leaders in 1935.[55] This came about as the result of a meeting between Millard and Dr Bardsley, Bishop of Leicester, in which they had discussed the religious aspect of euthanasia. Although Bardsley had registered an 'instinctive feeling' against the proposed Bill, he suggested that W. R. Matthews the Dean of St Paul's might be in sympathy with the Society's objectives. This was indeed the case, and Matthews suggested other figures who might be of a similar opinion. The resulting statement declared that in their opinion, voluntary euthanasia under the conditions outlined in the proposed Bill, should not be regarded as contrary to the teachings of Christ or the principles of Christianity.

In addition to this Millard was particularly keen to draw a distinction between legalised voluntary euthanasia and what was ordinarily understood by the term 'suicide'. This was understandable bearing in mind that suicide was cloaked by a number of negative connotations. It was a term which carried with it 'after centuries of condemnation, the stigma of a revolt against religion, law and public opinion'.[56]

Self-destruction in cases of incurable disease, however, had been subject to considerable support among some of the most eminent minds throughout history, as the welter of references cited by

Millard sought to demonstrate. 'Pliny declared that it was one of the greatest proofs of Providence that it has filled this world with herbs by which the weary may find a rapid and painless death.'[57] Seneca had also discussed the issue, stating that if he was able to choose between a torturous death and one that was easy, he would be inclined to select the latter. Of course disease should be endured if ultimately it could be cured, leaving the 'mind unimpaired ... But if I know that I will suffer for ever I will depart, not through fear of the pain but because it prevents all for which I would live.'[58] These were seemingly innocuous citations, but one is inclined to ask precisely what their purpose was. It would appear that for Millard, like many before him, ethical enlightenment lay in a reversion to past times.

Thomas More's *Utopia*, published in 1516, was also given considerable attention. Millard noted that while the inhabitants of More's imaginary kingdom sought effortlessly to restore the sick to health and to comfort the dying in their last hours, in the case of incurable and painful disease, patients were not only permitted, but actually encouraged to have their lives terminated. More was an able man noted for 'his integrity and moral courage'[59] and while it was acknowledged that the term Utopian referred to something which 'although desirable, is impracticable or visionary',[60] Millard suggested that More's proposals were not at all fanciful, indeed many were eminently sensible. The section quoted by Millard clearly indicates an abundance of humanitarian sentiment but there is one rather contentious aspect. The passage reads:

> if the disease be not only incurable, but also full of continual pain and anguish: then the priests and the magistrates exhort the man, seeing he is not able to do any duty of life, and by overliving his own death is noisome and irksome to others, and grievous to himself: that he will determine with himself no longer to cherish that pestilent and painful disease. And seeing that his life is to him but a torment, that he will not be unwilling to die, but rather take a good hope to him, and either dispatch himself out of that painful life as out of a prison, or a rack of torment, or else suffer to be rid out of it by other. And in so doing they tell him he shall do wisely, seeing by his death he shall lose no commodity, but end his pain. And because in that act he shall follow the counsel of the priests, that is to say, of the interpreters of God's will and pleasure, they show him that he shall do like a Godly and virtuous man ...[61]

It is the reference to a protracted death which is 'noisome and irksome to others' which appears to have caused considerable anxiety for the opponents of euthanasia.

Precisely the same quotation was cited by Lord Ponsonby of Shulbrede when introducing the Voluntary Euthanasia (Legalisation) Bill to the House of Lords.[62] It was also an issue which the Society as a whole failed to address satisfactorily. Millard had acknowledged that there was the 'question of possible abuse, e.g., by friends anxious for selfish reasons to rid themselves of a troublesome patient'[63] but suggested that this would not cause a problem as 'a permit could only be obtained where a man was suffering from a fatal disease'.[64] He was quite open about the issue, stating that in many cases the motive prompting the patient to opt for euthanasia would not only be the desire to avoid pain and suffering, but also the mental and physical strain inflicted upon one's 'nearest and dearest'. Viewed from this standpoint, euthanasia would come to be regarded as something heroic, an act of true altruism, to be applauded not deprecated.[65] Millard had also noted in his *Fortnightly Review* article, that those who desired to 'shirk' a painful and lingering death did so not only for 'themselves' but because of the 'strain and mental anguish which such an illness may entail upon those they love [which] may be an even greater dread'.[66] Evidently, the patient was not to be the sole beneficiary of euthanasia. Nevertheless, as opponents were quick to point out, pressure exerted either overtly or subliminally on a terminally-ill patient making them feel a burden might prompt them to choose euthanasia when ordinarily they would wish to die naturally. The suggestion that the patient's sense of being a burden might in part justify the application of euthanasia provides ample scope for the development of thin-end-of-the-wedge arguments.

Peculiarly for someone who was keen to put euthanasia in a class separate from suicide Millard appealed to the defenders of suicide to aid his advocacy of euthanasia. Moreover these examples failed to resolve the persistent ambiguity vis-à-vis altruism and the slippery slope. His citation of David Hume's essay *On Suicide* is particularly instructive. 'Suppose that it is no longer in my power to promote the interests of society; suppose that I am a burden to it; suppose that my life hinders some person from being much more useful to society. In such cases, my resignation of life must not only be innocent but laudable.'[67]

This was another example which Lord Ponsonby employed in

his unsuccessful advocacy in the Lords. From this extract, it would seem that in order to be worthwhile, a life must contribute something of value to society and should certainly not be a burden to it. Perhaps the Society was simply misguided in selecting texts which were inappropriate for the proposed legislative reform, and which served only to conflate a number of separate issues, but the ambiguity was left unresolved. Millard merely suggested that the most important distinguishing factor between euthanasia and suicide was the motive prompting the act. While suicide was often prompted by 'moral cowardice' with absolute disregard for the pain and suffering that this might cause others and should therefore be condemned, 'legalised voluntary euthanasia would come into quite a different category as an act which was rational, courageous, and often highly altruistic'.[68]

Occasionally, there was also a degree of flippancy to Millard's rhetoric, which aroused some concern. In an address to the British Medical Association Centenary Meeting, he turned to the question of possible abuse by friends and relatives who might wish a 'troublesome invalid out of the way. ... Well, Grandpa, if the pain is really as bad as you make out, I wonder you don't apply for euthanasia!'[69] Remarks of such a selfish and unfeeling nature might plausibly be made from time to time, and they would certainly cause mental distress. Evidently, Millard was not perturbed, 'one effect which such a remark, or even the possibility of it, would probably have is that it would make querulous old folk more careful how they dilated upon their aches and pains, and this might be a good thing for all concerned.'[70] While it seems likely that this statement was suffused with a hint of black humour, such sledgehammer sensitivity can have done little to sway the floating voter to the movement for voluntary euthanasia.

Millard persistently exposed himself to objection with his suggestion that euthanasia might be motivated by altruistic considerations. '[I]n many cases it would be prompted by considerations for others as much as by the desire to obtain relief from physical agony.'[71] He also cited the example of Captain Oates of the Scott Antarctic Expedition, who walked out of his tent knowing that he would be frozen to death, because as a sick man he was a burden to his fellow explorers. Noting that Oates was a 'very gallant gentleman', Millard posed the rhetorical question of whether anyone would regard his suicide as 'morally wrong'.[72] This was a rather ill-considered analogy. The extremities of choice in this case were entirely inappropriate for a comparison with voluntary euthanasia. Regardless of Dr Millard's intentions, allusions to societal burdens only served to stoke the fires of the opposition, with critics seeking to highlight the subliminal, non-medical pressures acting upon a patient to opt for euthanasia.

In fact from the outset it appears that Millard was perfectly alert to the problematic nature of the term euthanasia. This is immediately apparent from his Presidential Address in which he cited the *Encyclopaedia of Religion and Ethics*, which defined euthanasia as: 'The doctrine or theory that in certain circumstances when owing to disease, senility or the like, a person's life has permanently ceased to be either agreeable or useful, the sufferer should be painlessly killed either by himself or another.'[73]

Alongside the hedonistic form of euthanasia, this definition had alluded to euthanasia on the grounds of an individual's lack of utility. Seemingly aware of the term's elasticity, he had been quick to clarify precisely what he had in mind, and was quite explicit with regard to the proposed recipients of euthanasia. Despite the presence of Dr C. E. Goddard on the Voluntary Euthanasia Legalisation Society's Consultative Medical Council, Millard was not advocating 'anything beyond euthanasia for the dying where such a course is *expressly desired by the individual concerned*'.[74] In fact, direct reference was made to Goddard's paper of 1901 in which voluntary euthanasia had been juxtaposed with the proposal of euthanasia for particular cases of 'hopeless imbeciles, idiots and monstrosities'. It was noted that such a proposal raised a rather 'different and more difficult issue'. It was 'hardly surprising that Dr Goddard's paper, written as it was thirty years ago, was regarded as being too much in advance of public opinion.' In order to prevent confusion and 'misapprehension', Millard's Presidential Address made absolutely clear that his proposal did not include the mercy-killing of 'imbeciles and mental defectives'. The notion that old people who had become a burden to their families 'should be quietly consigned to the lethal chamber' was also rejected. Nor was he seeking to legalise or encourage a generalised form of suicide.

But as we have seen, ambiguity was never far away, and the merest hint of possible extensions to the Bill provided tactical liabilities. We might note that the *Sind Medical Journal* managed to get its facts hopelessly muddled and was under the impression that the

Voluntary Euthanasia (Legalisation) Bill would ensure that 'incurable imbeciles' would form the bulk of the 'Euthanasia murders'.[75] The article conceded that 'incurable imbeciles' were a considerable drag upon society, and that mental asylums were a definite burden upon the exchequer, but while it might be 'some gain to the public purse', it would not be of a substantial nature. 'Surely the states of the world are not so bankrupt economically or intellectually to devise and provide means to let these few people have their natural span of life'.[76]

Despite its manifest inaccuracy, and despite the fact that this was a rather obscure, non-British publication, the *Sind Medical Journal* was not alone in voicing concerns of this nature. A glance at the press in general, and the Catholic press in particular reveals the widespread prevalence of the slippery-slope argument. A letter to the editor of the *Leicester Mercury* entitled 'What next?' provides a particularly instructive example. 'Sir, Divorce, birth-control, sterilisation, and now euthanasia! My word, the old Pagan Rome would have had a lot to learn from us.'[77] At the annual conference of the Catholic Women's League in February 1932, Archbishop Downey (Roman Catholic Archbishop of Liverpool) summarised the situation as he saw it:

> under the aegis of education there is at the present time a craze for artificial interference with the laws of nature which is supposed to be demanded by modern enlightenment. We have recently been treated to a great deal of muddled thinking by eugenist reformers in a hurry. They are advocating, all in one breath, birth control, death control, euthanasia, life control and sterilisation. Apparently it is too much to expect that these alleged social reformers will consider the mere morality of what they are advocating.[78]

It is clear that Downey was conflating a number of different issues and probably intentionally. By lumping these concerns into one category he was depicting a concerted assault upon Divine Providence, which was decidedly imprecise. Nevertheless, one of the most obvious results of a prosopographical analysis of the Voluntary Euthanasia Legalisation Society is the high level of membership of the Eugenics Society. But, as we have seen, membership of the Eugenics Society by no means predisposed one to the advocacy of eugenic euthanasia. It is misleading to assume that allegiance to one organisation automatically ensured support for the other. Indeed, whilst Lord Horder was an active member of the Eugenics Society, he felt unable to support Millard's Bill and in fact spoke against it in the Lords' debate.

Nevertheless, Millard had enquired whether the Eugenics Society would be willing to include euthanasia in its Aims and Objects. This request was declined on the grounds that the eugenic implications of the proposed Bill were slight. As Dr C. P. Blacker, General Secretary of the Eugenics Society suggested, voluntary euthanasia for the terminally ill, which had much to commend it on humanitarian grounds, seemed to have no eugenic bearing. Euthanasia for a second group, 'children born with hereditary deformities which they are likely to transmit to posterity',[79] on the other hand, did have eugenic implications. But the number of such cases was thought to be limited, confined mainly to cases of gross skeletal deformities and certain forms of blindness. In such cases, eugenic sterilisation seemed to be a more appropriate course of action. Indeed, Millard concurred:

> If ultimately the measure were extended to include new-born children suffering from gross deformities, etc. the eugenic effect would still be very small, as this class of child is not very likely ever to become a parent. Apart from that, however I think it would be inadvisable to raise the issue at this juncture, either from the point of view of eugenics or euthanasia. It would certainly create much prejudice, and I can see no corresponding advantages.[80]

Whilst Millard had indicated that the Bill might be extended at a later date, he realised that it was only the 'right to die' not the 'right to kill' which had any *realistic* chance of being legalised at the present.[81]

Perhaps surprisingly, both Blacker and Millard had excluded the mentally defective from this possible second category. The Revd Dr R. F. Rattray, a member of the Executive Committee whom Millard had cited in his inaugural address to lend ecclesiastical weight to his proposals, did not. He advocated measures which can only have embarrassed his conservative colleagues. 'I go farther than Dr Millard, I think there is a strong case for euthanasia without the knowledge of the patient in the case of children suffering from hopeless and terrible torment, births of an abnormal kind. Surely it is not justified to prolong these lives, letting them be prey on normal people, undermining their health and sanity.'[82]

Rattray also spoke explicitly of extending euthanasia to the congenital idiot and imbecile.[83] Interestingly, Millard's response was less categorical than one might have assumed, 'desirable as this may be on purely humanitarian grounds it raises very special difficulties. I think that in the initial stages it would be better to confine euthanasia [to cases] where the patient himself expressly desires it.'[84] Nor was Rattray alone. An article appeared in the *Daily Herald* in March 1932 with the headline 'Lethal Chamber for Babies'.[85] This referred to a proposal put forward by Mr J. Myles Bickerton, Dean of the Royal Eye Hospital Southwark (a member of the Voluntary Euthanasia Legalisation Society's Consultative Medical Council) in an address to the Eugenics Society. Noting the increased incidence of blindness, he proposed to offer the parents of infants with gross defects an opportunity to end their child's life. In addition to raising philosophical concerns, there was a very practical dimension to these discussions. During the 1930s there were a number of high- profile legal cases which impinged directly upon these issues, most notable of which was the Brownhill case.

In December 1934 a Mrs Brownhill of Yorkshire was convicted for the murder of her thirty-year-old imbecile son Denis. Mrs Brownhill had devoted her life to caring for Denis, who was unable to do anything for himself. When she became ill and was required to go into hospital for a serious operation, she could not bear to see her son abandoned. Taking precipitate action, she gave Denis a large dose of aspirin to induce sleepiness and then placed a gas tube in his mouth, killing him. In his summing up Mr Justice Goddard remarked that:

> The time may come – we don't know – when it may be the law of this country that an imbecile, an idiot may be sent to a merciful death. That is not the law at the present time, and neither you nor I have the right to make laws. We have to take the law as it is, always remembering that in other and higher hands mercy may be extended. No person in this country has the right to take the life of any other human being because he or she thought it would be better for them to die.[86]

Sentence of death was passed, but the jury urged the 'strongest possible recommendation to mercy.' While the judge had no option in his sentencing, his remarks reveal sentiments expressed by many; the life of an imbecile was not of equal standing. This was certainly a step on from the form of euthanasia with which Killick Millard was principally concerned, but many were prepared to advocate such an extension. In an article dealing explicitly with this case, Havelock Ellis wrote: 'While we are all busily engaged, at vast expense, in preparing to kill off or torture the most promising citizens, even women and children, in the next war, we are terribly afraid of killing those citizens whom we all regard as financially unpromising.'[87]

This was perhaps the crudest example of its type. Havelock Ellis had in fact outlined his views more fully in a book published in 1931. He evidently regarded the prohibition of infanticide as 'one of the unfortunate results of Christianity'[88] and suggested further that 'there is a place in humanity for murder, that is to say by killing the unfit'.[89] It was 'Sisyphean' for a society to strive for social betterment while allowing 'entry into life ... more freely to the weak, the incompetent, and the defective than to the strong, the efficient, and the sane.'[90]

Such views were subject to the strongest criticism from the Catholic opposition. Dr Thomas Colvin a distinguished medical man, a Past Master of St Luke's Catholic Medical Guild, and a writer to the Catholic press on medico-social subjects, asked whether euthanasia would be:

> a triumph of might over right and the tyranny of the strong over the weak and feeble? Would it not deaden and destroy the finest and noblest feelings in man – pity and compassion for pain and suffering? ... would it not be putting back the hands of the clock of civilisation and a reversal to the law of the jungle, with nature red in tooth and claw?[91]

The Universe pursued this line by indicating that should this 'Bill to promote murder'[92] be passed, 'idiots', 'lunatics', and 'imbeciles' would be murdered. Dr Letitia Fairfield CBE, Senior Medical Officer, London County Council, a Roman Catholic who throughout the 1930s was a vehement opponent of sterilisation,[93] argued at the South London Catholic Citizens Parliament that the present-day standpoint on mental defectives appeared to be that because they contributed nothing of value to the world, their lives were 'utterly useless'. 'Surely it is much better that they should die, than live on, an incubus on others, and not useful in any way.'[94] The depiction of such crude utilitarian reasoning was not entirely misplaced.

No matter how firmly Millard might assert that his Bill was

concerned only with voluntary euthanasia,[95] thin-end of the wedge arguments were extremely difficult to suppress. This was particularly so when leading figures within the movement repeatedly made ambiguous or contradictory statements. Once the law permits the command 'Thou shalt not kill' to be broken, it is likely that the slope would become more and more slippery.[96] C. J. Bond for example, indicated that once the principle of voluntary euthanasia for incurable and painful disease had been established, 'it would be extended to other cases'.[97] Nor was Lord Moynihan immune from the occasional *faux pas*. Referring to the possibility of euthanasia for the 'defective', he suggested that 'if a child is born an idiot and there is not the slightest chance of recovery, then the question might be considered'.[98]

Indeed, these concerns surfaced in the Lords' debate in addition to the arguments for and against the more limited form of euthanasia. The Bill was introduced into the House by Lord Ponsonby owing to the death of Lord Moynihan, and one must feel a degree of sympathy for Millard, as Ponsonby's advocacy left much to be desired. Barristers across the country must have despaired when he remarked that: 'I go so far as to say that the consciousness of being a burden, the despairing view that you yourself are no longer of any use, the prolonged anxiety of others of which the patient is aware, may be as poignant as the suffering itself.'[99]

Prudent this was not. Ponsonby had in fact handed the opposition all the ammunition they required. Nor can he have allayed many fears when he suggested that 'we have restricted our proposals in this Bill purposely, whatever our views may be about Mongolians, congenital idiots and senile dementia, where safeguards would have to be very much more strict and where there would be no doubt other great difficulties'.[100] This merely succeeded in revealing the inflationary scope of the Bill.

Both Lord Horder and the Archbishop of Canterbury were clearly concerned. Horder registered his surprise at the stress given to the patient's consciousness of being a burden 'as being important – even, the noble Lord said, the most important condition for legalised euthanasia'.[101] Referring to the inflationary potential, the Archbishop of Canterbury said that while he was not normally impressed by 'thin end of the wedge' arguments 'we cannot dismiss from our minds the fact that many of those who are behind the noble Lord in bringing forward this Bill definitely contemplate its after-extension to other cases which for the present he has ruled out. He says that this Bill is merely to unlock the door, but if the door is once unlocked it will soon be opened wide.'[102] This seems to have been a perfectly reasonable observation.

Although euthanasia was debated in the House of Lords it does not appear to have been a party-political issue. Indeed, discussion of politics has been conspicuous by its absence from this chapter. Ministry of Health files reveal that the subject was discussed in governmental circles, but it was considered to be a controversial issue from which 'no benefit to mental or physical health' could result and as such Government support for the proposed Bill was out of the question. Euthanasia was said to be a matter 'outside the proper range of Government intervention and to be one which should be left to the conscience of the individual members of the House.'[103]

This chapter has sought to show that an adequate explanation of the failure to obtain legislation on voluntary euthanasia must take into account objections centring on the altruistic and norma-tive aspects of euthanasia. Both aspects had featured prominently in the rhetoric of the Voluntary Euthanasia Legalisation Society over the preceding five years and had done much to foster the slip-pery-slope argument. The examination of the Society's membership has shown that the euthanasia movement was a collection of diverse individuals motivated by strong humanitarian sentiment. The high proportion of progressive, reformist individu-als, particularly from within the medical profession would seem to indicate that the Society was very much a product of its time. We have also seen that while the eugenic dimension of euthanasia which had been so prominent during the immediate post-war years was largely eclipsed, a complex relationship persisted between eugenic ideas and the question of euthanasia. This contributed to the anxieties voiced by the opponents of the legali-sation of voluntary euthanasia. In emphasising the centrality of concerns about non-voluntary euthanasia in securing the defeat of the 1936 Voluntary Euthanasia (Legalisation) Bill, this chapter has attempted to rectify the imbalance evident in preceding accounts. Nevertheless, it must be stressed that this was only one aspect of a complex of objections which included opposition to changing the

physician's ethos, and various practical objections such as the accu
racy of terminal diagnoses. It is of course clear that opposition from
within the medical profession was crucially important in the defeat
of the Bill. Lord Dawson had suggested that even if the practice
were legalised, 'the law remain nugatory'. However, we might like
to note Dawson's remark to the effect that the legalisation of voluntary euthanasia 'would deter those who are, as I think, carrying out
their mission of mercy'.[104] This was a rather peculiar argument
which seemed to praise a paternalistic yet illegal practice. Dawson
also seemed to miss the crux of the Bill, namely that it was
designed to allow patients to *request* euthanasia. In fact this
eminent medical authority who was so important to the defeat of
the Bill also happened to be rather instrumental in affecting a 'good
death' for George V, as his Sandringham notebook reveals.

> At about 11 o'clock it was evident that the last stage might endure
> for many hours, unknown to the Patient but little comporting with
> that dignity and serenity which he so richly merited and which
> demanded a brief final scene, Hours of waiting just for the mechan-
> ical end when all that is really life has departed only exhausts the
> onlookers and keeps them so strained that they cannot avail them-
> selves of the solace of thought, communion or prayer. I therefore
> decided to determine the end and injected (myself) morphia gr.3/4
> & shortly afterwards cocaine gr.1 into the distended jugular
> vein ...[105]

Despite the vocal opposition to euthanasia among particular physicians, it would seem that a strong notion of medical paternalism
sanctioned the surreptitious employment of this procedure.

Notes

1 The Society has changed its name at various times being known as the
  Voluntary Euthanasia Legalisation Society, the Euthanasia Society, EXIT,
  and currently the Voluntary Euthanasia Society.
2 *Public Health*, Nov. 1931, pp. 39–47; *BMJ*, 24 Oct. 1931, p. 754.
3 The gentleman in question was Mr O. W. Greene (Obituary, *The Times*, 14
  Mar. 1935, p. 15) who had initially offered to give the Society a sum in the
  region of £10,000 but subsequently retracted this offer of financial support
  because he would not consent to the view that a patient must be suffering
  from an incurable condition in order for euthanasia to be justified. See
  Voluntary Euthanasia Legalisation Society Archives, Contemporary
  Medical Archives Centre, Wellcome Institute, Euston Road, London, here-
  after CMAC/SA/VES. Minutes of the Society CMAC/SA/VES/A.1, Minutes of
  9 Apr. 1935 and 18 Sep. 1935. Greene made no provision for the Society in

his will. See CMAC/SA/VES/A.2, Minutes of 4 Mar. 1936.

4 CMAC/SA/VES/A.1, Minutes of 14 Feb. 1935.

5 See Millard obituaries: *Public Health*, Apr. 1952, p. 123; *BMJ*, 22 Mar. 1952, p. 661; *The Lancet*, 22 Mar. 1952, p. 619.

6 C. Killick Millard, *The Vaccination Question in the Light of Modern Experience* (London, 1914); *Medical Officer*, 21 May 1927, p. 241.

7 *Medical Officer*, 16 Jun. 1918, p. 195.

8 *Medical Officer*, 23 Feb. 1918, p. 58.

9 *Medical Officer*, 4 Jun. 1921, p.245.

10 *Medical Officer*, 4 Jan. 1919, p. 7.

11 *Medical Officer*, 23 Nov. 1918, p. 179.

12 This was the theme of Millard's speech at Marie Stopes's Queen's Hall Meeting, May 1921. See Keith Briant, *Marie Stopes: A Biography* (London, 1962) pp. 145–6.

13 *Medical Officer*, 23 Nov. 1918, p. 179.

14 Richard Soloway, *Demography and Degeneration, Eugenics and the Declining Birthrate in Twentieth Century Britain* (London, 1990) p. 176.

15 *Ibid.*

16 Charles Killick Millard, 'Contraception and the Medical Officer of Health', *Journal of State Medicine*, Jan. 1931, pp. 46–54.

17 CMAC/SA/VES C.4 *Summary of an Address on the Life and Work of Charles John Bond*, by Lt Col Sir Robert Martin.

18 See, C. J. Bond, *On the Nature and Meaning of Evil and Suffering as Seen from the Evolutionary Standpoint* (Leicester, 1937) p. 19.

19 John Macnicol, 'Eugenics and the campaign for voluntary sterilisation in Britain between the wars', *Social History of Medicine*, Vol. 2, No. 2, (1989) p. 165.

20 CMAC/SA/VES/A.1 Address by Mr C. J. Bond to a meeting of the Leicester Socroptomists' Club, 31 Mar. 1935.

21 *Who Was Who*, 1996, A. & C. Black (Publishers) Ltd, CD Rom.

22 In 1931 Rattray became Minister of the Memorial Church (Unitarian) Cambridge.

23 Greta Jones, *Social Hygiene in Twentieth-Century Britain* (London, 1986).

24 See Dorothy Porter, 'Enemies of the race: biologism, environmentalism, and public health in Edwardian England', *Victorian Studies*, Winter 1991, Vol. 34, pp. 159–78.

25 See: G. R. Searle, 'Eugenics and politics in Britain in the 1930s', *Annals of Science*, Vol. 36, 1979.

26 C. Killick Millard, 'The case for euthanasia', *Fortnightly Review*, Dec. 1931, p. 718.

27 Tim Helme, 'The Voluntary Euthanasia (Legalisation) Bill (1936) revisited', *Journal of Medical Ethics*, 17, 1991, pp. 25–9.

28 *Public Health*, p. 39.

29 Statistics from the Registrar General cited in Millard, 'The case for euthanasia', p. 701.

30 *Ibid.*, p. 704.

31 See *On the State of Public Health. Annual Report of the Chief Medical Officer of the Ministry of Health for the Year 1927* (London, 1928) p. 102.

32 See *Medical Officer*, 19 Jan. 1929, p. 28.

33 *Chief Medical Officer's Annual Report*, p. 99.

34 CMAC/SA/VES/B.3 *Evening Standard*, 25 Oct. 1935.
35 Millard, 'The case for euthanasia'.
36 CMAC/SA/VES/C.3 Leicester Evening Mail, 17 Oct. 1931.
37 See, Jonathan Glover, *Causing Death and Saving Lives* (London, [1977], 1990) pp. 92–110.
38 *Public Health*, Nov. 1931, p. 39.
39 *House of Lords Debates* (*H.L. Deb.*), 1 Dec. 1936, c. 480.
40 CMAC/SA/VES/B.3 Letter to the editor, *The Lancet*, 21 Nov. 1935 from A. S. Lundell Bankart.
41 *The Lancet*, 21 Nov. 1936, p. 1215.
42 CMAC/SA/VES/A.12 The Voluntary Euthanasia (Legalisation) Bill 1936.
43 *H.L. Deb.* Voluntary Euthanasia (Legalisation) Bill, 1 Dec. 1936, c. 492.
44 CMAC/SA/VES/C.3 Extract from an address by Dr C. Killick Millard at the British Medical Association Centenary Meeting, 28 July 1932.
45 CMAC/SA/VES/B.2 *Sunday Express*, 13 Oct. 1931.
46 CMAC/SA/VES/B.3 *The Universe, The Catholic Newspaper*, 26 Oct. 1934.
47 'Norfolk Branch: West Norfolk Division: discussion on voluntary euthanasia', *BMJ*, p. 279.
48 *Public Health*, Nov. 1931, p. 40.
49 CMAC/SA/VES/B.11 *Catholic Medical Journal*, p. 75.
50 CMAC/SA/VES/C.3 Extract from the *Leicester Evening Mail*, 28 July 1932 regarding a paper delivered by Dr Millard on 'The medico-legal aspect of voluntary euthanasia' at the British Medical Association Conference on the same day.
51 *Public Health*, Nov. 1931, pp. 42–3.
52 CMAC/SA/VES/C.3 *Leicester Evening Mail*, 27 Oct. 1931.
53 CMAC/SA/VES/C.3 *Leicester Evening Mail*, 17 Oct. 1931.
54 *Ibid.*
55 CMAC/SA/VES/A.13 This statement was signed by the following: Peter Green, Canon of Manchester, Rural Dean of Salford; W. R. Matthews, Dean of St Paul's; R. D. A. Major, Principal, Ripon Hall, Oxford; F. R. C. Payne, Canon Chancellor of Leicester; J. M. Creed, Ely Professor of Divinity, Cambridge, Canon of Ely; Harold Anson, Master of the Temple, Canon of Southwark; W. R. Inge, Ex-Dean of St Paul's; Charles E. Raven, Regius Professor of Divinity, Cambridge, Canon of Ely; H. R. L. Sheppard, Canon of St Paul's, Ex-Dean of Canterbury, Ex-Vicar of St Martin-in-the-Fields; C. F. Russell, Headmaster, Merchant Taylors' School, Crosby; H. Wheeler Robinson, Principal, Regent's Park College; T. Rhondda Williams, Chairman, Congregational Union; F. W. Norwood, Minister, City Temple; E. C. Hewlett Johnson, Dean of Canterbury; Revd A. Herbert-Gray, well-known Presbyterian divine, author of several books on religious and social subjects.
56 Public Health, Nov. 1931, p. 40.
57 *Ibid.*, p. 40.
58 *Ibid.*, p. 41.
59 *Ibid.*, p. 40.
60 *Ibid.*
61 Extract from More's *Utopia*, cited by Millard, *Public Health*, Nov. 1931, p. 40.
62 *H.L. Deb.* c. 470.
63 *Public Health*, Nov. 1931, p. 46.

64 *Ibid.*
65 *Ibid.*
66 Millard, 'The case for euthanasia', p. 701.
67 *Public Health*, Nov. 1931, p. 43.
68 *Ibid.*, pp. 43–4.
69 *Ibid.*
70 *Ibid.*
71 CMAC/SA/VES/C.3 *Leicester Evening Mail*, 17 Oct. 1931.
72 Millard, 'The case for euthanasia', p. 701.
73 *Public Health*, Nov. 1931, p. 39.
74 *Fortnightly Review*, Dec. 1931, pp. 704–5.
75 CMAC/SA/VES/C.4 Editorial, *Sind Medical Journal*, Dec. 1935 (Karachi).
76 *Ibid.*, pp. 144–5.
77 CMAC/SA/VES/B.2 *Leicester Mercury*, 31 Oct. 1931.
78 CMAC/SA/VES/B.3 *The Catholic Herald*, 6 Feb. 1932.
79 Archives of the Eugenics Society, Contemporary Medical Archives Centre, Wellcome Institute for the History of Medicine (CMAC/EUG). CMAC/EUG/C.232 Correspondence between Dr C. Killick Millard and Dr C. P. Blacker, 11 Feb. 1935.
80 CMAC/EUG/C.232 Correspondence between Millard and Blacker, 9 Sept. 1935.
81 CMAC/EUG/C.232 Correspondence between Millard and Blacker n. d.
82 CMAC/SA/VES/B.2 *Cambridge Chronicle*, 21 Mar. 1934.
83 CMAC/SA/VES/B.3 *Leicester Evening Mail*, 6 Oct. 1934.
84 *Ibid.*
85 CMAC/SA/VES/B.3 *Daily Herald*, 16 Mar. 1932.
86 CMAC/SA/VES/B.3 Cited in the *Daily Mail*, 1 Nov. 1934.
87 CMAC/SA/VES/C.4 Article by Havelock Ellis for the American press, 7 Dec. 1934.
88 Havelock Ellis, More essays of love and virtue, (London, 1931) p. 1777, cited in a review article by W. R. Inge, *The Eugenics Review* 1931–32, Vol. 23, p. 264.
89 *Ibid.*
90 Cited in Daniel J. Kevles, *In the Name of Eugenics: Genetics and the Uses of Human Heredity* (New York, 1985) p. 92.
91 CMAC/SA/VES/B.3 *The Universe, The Catholic Newspaper*, 26 Oct. 1934.
92 CMAC/SA/VES/B.3 This term was coined by Bishop Brown, cited in *The Universe* 29 Nov. 1935.
93 See Greta Jones, *Social Hygiene*, p. 91.
94 CMAC/SA/VES/B.3 *The Universe*, 29 Nov. 1935.
95 CMAC/SA/VES/B.3 In a letter to the *BMJ*, 28 Nov. 1935, Millard stated explicitly that lunatics and mental defectives were deliberately excluded from the scope of his Bill.
96 CMAC/SA/VES/B.5 *BMJ*, 11 Jan. 1936, Letter from Robert A. Fleming of the Royal Hospital for Incurables, Edinburgh.
97 CMAC/SA/VES/B.3 *Daily Mail*, 11 Nov. 1935.
98 CMAC/SA/VES/B.3 *Evening Standard*, 25 Oct. 1935.
99 *H.L. Deb.* c. 469.
100 *Ibid.*, c. 471.
101 *Ibid.*, c. 493.

102 *Ibid.*, c. 488.
103 Public Record Office (PRO) PRO/MH/58/95018/8/42A. Nov. 1936 Euthanasia, Voluntary Euthanasia Legalisation Bill.
104 *Ibid.*, c. 485.
105 Extract cited in Francis Watson, 'The death of George V', *History Today*, Vol. 36, 1986, p. 28.

5

'Euthanasia' and mental defectives: the British euthanasia movement and the impact of the Nazi euthanasia programme, 1936–50

The reform which the Voluntary Euthanasia Legalisation Society sought to effect was a 'radical departure from olde-established custom and tradition'[1] and it came as little surprise that the Society was confronted by strong opposition. But, despite the defeat of the 1936 Voluntary Euthanasia (Legalisation) Bill, a widespread debate had taken place during the five years since Dr Charles Killick Millard had raised the question in his presidential address to the Society of Medical Officers of Health. This ensured that considerable sympathy had been aroused and an influential body of opinion had been attracted to the movement in favour of voluntary euthanasia. In the circumstances the Lords' defeat was thought to have provided little cause for discouragement. As the Society's ethical statement demonstrated, considerable progress had been made in combating theological obstacles. It was deemed 'important and significant' that the Archbishop of Canterbury had not opposed the Bill on religious grounds, because 'hitherto, the religious objection' had 'been for many a serious difficulty'.[2] Bearing in mind the relatively small expenditure at the Society's disposal, it was clear that much progress had been made in bringing this previously obscure issue into the forum of public debate. Indeed, the tenor of the Society's first annual report was generally optimistic. A great deal of work would be required in order to educate public opinion before a second Bill could be introduced with any realistic chance of success, but this was thought to be eminently feasible.

Yet, it was not until 1950 that the Society managed to bring the issue before the House of Lords for a second time, when Lord Chorley of Kendal, a Vice-President of the Society, introduced a motion which called attention to the need to legalise voluntary euthanasia. This procedure had been considered a 'better' and

'simpler' method for furthering the cause rather than the reintro-
duction of a Voluntary Euthanasia (Legalisation) Bill.[3] It would
seem that the Society was conscious that the prevailing moral
climate rendered legislative success at this juncture highly unlikely.
The motion was certainly greeted with far more hostility than Lord
Ponsonby's venture of 1936. Indeed, the opposition was so overwhelming that the motion was withdrawn without forcing a
division of the House. The strength of opposition was demonstrated
further when in 1950 the World Medical Association adopted a resolution which recommended that national medical associations
should 'condemn the practice of euthanasia in any circumstance'.[4]
In the same year the British Medical Association endorsed this resolution.[5]

It would take a further nineteen years before the Society was
again able to present a Voluntary Euthanasia Legalisation Bill to
Parliament. Throughout the intervening period, the British
euthanasia movement found itself under an extremely dark cloud,
oppressed by seemingly insurmountable objections. The chronol-
ogy of this period and the focus of this chapter thus bridges the
comparative optimism of 1936 and the absolute despondency of
1950. It documents the intervening years which were perhaps the
most tumultuous in the history of the British euthanasia movement,
and suggests that the revelations of the Nazi euthanasia programme
effectively precluded legislative reform of euthanasia for the fore-
seeable future. The circumstances in which the House of Lords
debate of 1950 took place differed entirely from those of 1936. The
debate of this period was heavily conditioned by images of the Nazi
programme of non-voluntary euthanasia; an illegal operation which
operating in successive stages from 1939 throughout the war years
was responsible for the covert killing of approximately 100,000 liber-
ally-defined defectives. Although it will be necessary to make
frequent reference to the Nazi euthanasia programme, such reference will be made only to the extent to which it sheds light on, or
was an integral part of the British euthanasia movement. The
German programme had its own inordinate complexities which
could not be explored in any detail here, and for which a substantial
secondary literature already exists.[6]

In the period immediately following the defeat of the Voluntary
Euthanasia (Legalisation) Bill of 1936 numerous eminent figures
within the Voluntary Euthanasia Legalisation Society began to

speak more openly about the application of euthanasia to defectives. Even after the revelations of the Nazi euthanasia programme, reactions in Britain were far from uniform. While some historians have alluded to 'the wish to react against what happened in Germany'[7] this chapter suggests that this was only one of several reactions. It is possible to identify numerous advocates of non-voluntary euthanasia in a British context. This applied to the Voluntary Euthanasia Legalisation Society itself, to the broader populace, and to particular individuals active in the field of mental health care. A recent study of the problem of mental deficiency in England[8] has suggested that the Second World War led to an increasingly sympathetic attitude towards the disabled. Indicative of this was the heightened criticism of the conditions prevailing in the nation's mental hospitals and of 'discrimination against the mentally ill'.[9] Such a shift reflected 'libertarian concern over wrongful confinement of high-grade defectives'. It has also been observed, however, that 'there was far less interest in the seriously handicapped, who continued to be viewed as objects for paternal care not as possessors of rights'.[10] The evidence surveyed in this chapter certainly supports the view that low-grade defectives continued to receive little attention, but suggests further, that when these individuals were discussed, Draconian proposals which bore close similarities to the Nazi concept of destroying 'life unworthy of life' could be elicited.

Preaching before the University of Oxford on 7 March 1937, Dr E. W. Barnes, the Bishop of Birmingham and a signatory of the Voluntary Euthanasia Legalisation Society's ethical statement, had argued that 'the cost of social derelicts' and in particular the 'feeble-minded' was 'harmful in that indirectly' it pressed upon 'all classes'. He also believed that it was not right 'to keep alive individuals whom doctors know to be doomed from birth to a sub-human existence', and claimed that a 'false humanitarianism' was 'at the present a definite drag on social progress'.[11] This was a classic example of the way in which a multiplicity of motives were often advanced in favour of non-voluntary euthanasia for defectives. Clearly there was a concern with the incidence of mental deficiency, which was deemed to be both undesirable and economically disadvantageous, but allied to this was a belief that a life lacking particular mental characteristics was sub-human. In keeping such beings alive man was acting in a counter-selective and inhumane fashion, sponsoring the survival of that which was not fit to survive

While it seems incontrovertible that these motives were distinct from those prompting the more mainstream proposals for voluntary euthanasia, it is interesting to note that Killick Millard regarded the Bishop's remarks as very important. Although the case depicted would 'not quite' come within the scope of the Bill for voluntary euthanasia, it had 'an important bearing on the subject, and coming from a person in so high a place' was a 'distinctly encouraging sign'.[12] Barnes was certainly not the most conservative of ecclesiastics. He was a strong supporter of evolutionary ideas and a strong advocate of negative eugenic policies.[13] During the 1940s he would become the most outspoken advocate of non-voluntary euthanasia.

Mr C. J. Bond, Chairman and co-founder of the Voluntary Euthanasia Legalisation Society also remarked that he did not regard all human life as equally 'valuable or sacred'. Bond posed the question of how one could 'suppose that the life of a poor little mentally deficient child was as valuable as the life of a hard-working respectable and industrious citizen?' He was of the opinion that one should measure the 'value of human life' in terms of the 'capacity for happiness, joy, self-development and service to others'.[14] Once again we can see how the belief in the sub-human character of the mentally defective could be fused with an economic rationale for their destruction. In this regard we might note that the Mental Deficiency Act of 1913 had classified grades of mental defect in terms of social efficiency, and this might go some way to explaining why it was so common to find discussion of mental deficiency threaded with economic rhetoric.

The following year discussions pertaining to the non-voluntary killing of defectives gained practical bearing when euthanasia hit the headlines again. The catalyst was the trial of Mrs Kathleen Mumford a forty-year-old housewife accused of the 'mercy murder' of her five-year-old mentally defective son. Derek Mumford was incapable of doing a great deal for himself and had been pronounced an incurable imbecile. 'His legs were stiff. His right arm was paralysed and he could not even hold a cup properly.'[15] Having asked a doctor to terminate her son's life, and having had her request turned down, Mrs Mumford took the law into her own hands, held a gas tube to the boy's face until he was dead and then carried his body to the police station. Kathleen Mumford was sentenced to death, but expressed no regret, she said calmly, that while she was guilty in the eyes of the law, she believed that in the eyes of God she was not guilty. She went on to express thanks to the doctors whom she knew would have given her boy 'brains' if they had been able. But, there was no cure and as far as she was concerned, her child had nothing to live for, '[a]ll the days of his life he would have been an imbecile'. She ended the child's suffering and in so doing claimed to have acted in her son's best interests; 'as God would not take him away, I thought it my duty to help'.[16] Although Mrs Mumford was sentenced to death, the jury added 'the very strongest recommendation to mercy' and she was released quickly.

The fact that the *Daily Sketch* reported that this case had started a new nation-wide right-to-die campaign, illustrates how easy and common it was to confuse or conflate the concept of voluntary euthanasia with the application of non-voluntary euthanasia to mental defectives. This impression was reinforced by the comments of Dr F. W. Norwood, the ex-pastor of the City Temple. Using this opportunity to press for a re-examination of the problem of voluntary euthanasia, Norwood, who was also a signatory of the Voluntary Euthanasia Legalisation Society's ethical statement, argued rather misguidedly that, 'The point in the present case is that the dilemma of Mrs Mumford brings home the necessity for ... reconsideration of the legal right to kill.'[17] Even the more diplomatic Millard left the issue somewhat hazy when he stated that while Mrs Mumford's case was not one where the Society would have 'recommended euthanasia for the child ... the tragic circumstances have focused public attention on the problem'.[18]

It is interesting to note, however, that such remarks appear to have had little adverse affect upon the Society's fortunes. By the time of its third annual report, the Society was contemplating the re-introduction of a Voluntary Euthanasia Legalisation Bill in autumn 1939. The report concluded with the upbeat claim that the movement had 'come to stay'. What had once been the 'Utopian' dream of a handful of 'idealists' was now attracting increasing numbers of people 'including leaders' from all spheres of life. There was some uncertainty regarding the length of time it would take to pass legislation because much work remained to be done in educating public opinion, in removing misapprehension, and in combating opposition. Not everyone would live to see the ultimate victory, but they could be content in the knowledge that they were engaged in laying the foundations of a 'great reform' which might one day 'be regarded as marking an epoch in the history of civilisation. This is a humanitarian age, and ours is nothing if not a humanitarian movement.'[19]

However, 1939 proved to be a rather frustrating year. The Society's typist was commandeered for public duties and it was thought sensible to postpone work until the 'shock caused by the outbreak of war had somewhat subsided'.[20] During this period of comparative inactivity the primary objective of the Society had been to obtain new names for its list of 'Distinguished Supporters', and in this endeavour it was rather successful. In the course of 1939 the list had grown to some 400 names. The following year this had risen by another 400 names,[21] and by the end of 1941 by a further 150.[22] The Society was also able to report that a poll conducted by the British Institute of Public Opinion on the question, 'Should those suffering from an incurable disease be allowed the option under proper medical safeguards, of a voluntary death?' had recorded 62 per cent in favour, 22 per cent against, and 16 per cent had no opinion. Further analysis had indicated that neither age, sex nor economic status made any 'appreciable difference' to the answers volunteered.[23] Millard was also of the opinion that the effects of war might prove to be beneficial for the movement. The First World War was deemed to have altered considerably 'our whole outlook on life' and the present conflict could cause 'old standards' to be modified, 'old prejudices' to be swept away and 'new ideas' to be 'more readily accepted'.[24] The annual report for 1940 suggested that when the Society next brought its Bill before Parliament, which would not be until after the war, it would be in a much stronger position to command a hearing than had been the case in 1936. While the Society's optimism was not entirely misplaced, the events of the next year would prove to be rather destabilising to say the least.

Although British intelligence had received information regarding the Nazi destruction of mentally defective and infirm patients in 1940,[25] news of the Nazi euthanasia programme did not filter into the British press until the following year. One of the first papers to develop early reports about executions of the old and unfit was the *Daily Mirror*. It reported that the *Acta Apostolicae Sedis*, 'the Vatican publication in which the Pope outlines the policies that his Bishops are to follow', had published a reply to a question relating to the Nazi practice of 'euthanasia' posed by an unnamed German bishop.

Under the heading 'Concerning the direct killing of the innocent done by order of public authority' it was reported that the Supreme Sacred Congregation had been asked 'whether by order of public authority' it was 'licit directly to kill those who although they have committed no crime deserving death, yet, because of mental or physical or defects, are no longer able to benefit the nation, and are considered rather to burden the nation and obstruct its energy and strength'.[26] The Supreme Sacred Congregation held on Wednesday, 27 November 1940, had replied 'in the negative, since it is contrary to natural and divine positive law.'[27] The article reported that in September, October and November, 1940, 85,000 unfit people had been murdered in accordance with the 'Nazi doctrine which prescribes that any person, by reason of mental or physical defects, who can no longer be considered an asset to the State, is an enemy of the State'.[28] They were killed by means of carbon monoxide gas.

Seven days after this article appeared, the Voluntary Euthanasia Legalisation Society held its annual meeting in Leicester. There was no mention of the Nazi euthanasia programme. Millard remarked merely that the Society was in a stronger position than had been the case in 1936 and would endeavour to introduce a Bill after the war. Opponents of euthanasia, however, were not slow to add the revelations to their armoury. A letter to the *Leicester Mercury* provides a striking example: 'It was with grief and disgust that I read in your issue of Wednesday evening of the progress made by the Voluntary Euthanasia Legalisation Society. Are we to popularise the diabolical methods of Nazi Germany?'[29] Such conflation was not uncommon.

During September the publication of the fourth article from William Shirer's 'Berlin Diary' in the *Daily Express* exposed further details about the scope of Nazi 'euthanasia' atrocities. News was revealed about the removal and execution of the mentally deficient population of the Reich. Three possible motives were mooted, two of which seemed unlikely. The first was that they were carried out in order to save food. But bearing in mind that Germany was experiencing no acute food shortage, and that the removal of 100,000 persons was unlikely to make any significant difference in a country of eighty million, this motive seemed untenable. The second motive, that the killings were the product of experimentation with new poisonous gases and death rays, was considered possible though unlikely. While it was recognised that poison gases may have been used 'in putting these unfortunates out of the way   the experi-mentation was only incidental'.[30] The third motive was deemed the most likely, namely that the asylum killings were 'simply the result of the extreme Nazis deciding to carry out their sociological ideas'.[31] This was indeed the primary motive, justified in part by allusions to what Shirer cited as a fourth motive: 'They say the Nazis calculate that for every three or four institutional cases there must be one healthy German to look after them. This takes several thousand Germans away from more profitable employment. If the insane are killed off, it is argued by the Nazis there will be plenty of hospital space for the war wounded should the war be prolonged and large casualties occur. It's a Nazi messy business.'[32] The identification of crude utilitarian, economic and eugenic motivations was extremely accurate.

Recent research has shown that the explanations for the Nazi programme are complex, but it is clear that the ideological and intel-lectual climates from which they derived were not solely a product of the National Socialists' tenure of power. In a similar fashion to Great Britain, Germany had enjoyed a vibrant discussion about euthanasia in its many guises from the late nineteenth century onwards.[33] In the 1890s, polemicist Adolf Jost had modified the prevailing view of euthanasia as a dignified and 'gentle' death, by questioning the doctor's absolute obligation to maintain life. He argued not only in favour of voluntary euthanasia, but spoke also of 'negative human worth'. Such a concept sought to highlight the burden incurred by families and society as a whole, in addition to the misery and negative quality of life endured by the terminally-ill patient. Jost also argued that it was legitimate to terminate the lives of mentally handicapped individuals, whether they were capable of expressing the desire to end their life or not. Clearly the sentiments which had been voiced in Britain during the 1870s and which were examined in the first chapter of this book, held a considerable degree of international currency.

We might also note that in 1913 a draft law sanctioning euthanasia had been proposed by a terminally-ill patient suffering from lung disease; a draft law which was remarkably similar to Millard's Bill of 1936.[34] Perhaps the most influential German work on euthanasia, however, was Binding and Hoche's *Permission for the Destruction of Life Unworthy of Life* (*Die Freigabe der Vernichtung Lebens unwerten Lebens*), to which attention was drawn in Chapter 3.

Binding and Hoche proposed the legalisation of euthanasia for both terminally-ill *compos mentis* patients and for the *non compos mentis*. There was a strong economic rationale underpinning this text. The economic vicissitudes of the 1920s had fostered a considerable increase in the asylum population, which in turn placed a heavier burden upon the state. In such circumstances the idea of dividing patients between the curable and incurable, and utilising 'productive' patients within the asylum economy gained ground. Euthanasia for the incurably insane and hopelessly defective was thus identified as a mechanism for cost cutting.

Also at the core of Binding and Hoche's proposal was a belief that one could justifiably kill those lacking the essential mental qualities which rendered existence 'human'. We have already identified sentiments of a similar nature amongst such individuals as Lionel Tollemache, Annie Besant, F. W. Newman, C. E. Goddard, F. A. W. Gisborne, and C. J. Bond in a British context.

Despite these similarities, it is clear that the Nazi programme was seen as part and parcel of an overarching plan of racial purification. This was a peculiarly German phenomenon. In *Mein Kampf*, Hitler had remarked upon the need to make 'a new and ruthless choice according to strength and health'.[35] At the Nuremberg rally of 1929 he had also stated that if Germany were to add one million children per year and remove '700–800,000 of the weakest people then the final result might even be an increase in strength'. Hitler claimed that as a consequence of 'modern sentimental humanitarianism' Germany was attempting to 'maintain the weak at the expense of the healthy'.[36] 'Health and fertility became identified with German nationalism, and as a consequence changes in nationalism fed back into medicine and biology'.[37] But, even within the National Socialist state, at the level of rhetoric at least, non-voluntary euthanasia for defectives was justified on the grounds of relieving the suffering of individuals unable to request euthanasia themselves. As in all varieties of euthanasia, an ostensible assessment was to be made about when a particular life lacked a set of characteristics which made life worthy of being lived.

Indeed, we should note that although there were long-term ideological roots, the children's euthanasia programme begun in 1939 was said to have been precipitated by the case of a grossly defective infant whose parents requested that their baby should be killed mercifully. Hitler consented to the killing of the 'Knauer' baby, a baby which had deformed limbs and may have been both blind and an 'idiot'. This case has been seen as the 'pretext' which enabled the Führer to implement the euthanasia programme which he had envisaged much earlier; a programme which would kill children afflicted with physical and mental defects.[38] In no way is this meant as an apology for the Nazi euthanasia programme and a clear distinction must be made between the professed motivations of defendants at the Nuremberg Medical Trial and the practice of the programme which was so crude in its identification of victims, involving no physical examination of patients, and which included patients with such slight afflictions as a hair-lip. But, it must be recognised that several of the motivating factors which drove the Nazi programme were evident in Britain. Proposals for administering euthanasia to the mentally defective and insane had been persistent features of the euthanasia debate in Great Britain, and similar discussions were also evident in other countries.[39]

However, in both the children's euthanasia programme and the subsequent adult programme, many of the victims suffered from physical as opposed to mental disabilities. The 'criteria for inclusion in the pool' were similar to those which had been employed in the sterilisation programme. Thus, among those who were killed, we find individuals who suffered not from mental defect, but who were blind, deaf, mute, or had learning difficulties. While those who killed such patients may have 'rationalized that these patients were like animals who neither recognized nor cared for their environment; in fact ... the majority of patients killed were "orderly and conscious" and were "worthy persons"'.[40] Indeed, it is absolutely clear that one of the key criteria for inclusion in the programme was economic rather than medical.

Revealing as Shirer's account of the euthanasia programme was, perhaps the most important item of news concerned the preaching of a sermon by Clemens August Count von Galen, the Bishop of Münster. Von Galen drew attention to reports regarding the forcible removal of patients from sanatoria and asylums for the insane. Shortly afterwards the relatives had been informed of the unexpected death of their loved ones. There was a 'suspicion bordering on certainty' that this cluster of 'unexpected' deaths among the insane was no mere coincidence. They were brought about intentionally in accordance with the view that the lives of persons deemed 'unworthy to live' could be killed justifiably if they were of no 'use to the nation and State'. 'According to the judgment of some doctor, according to the opinion of some commission, they have become "unworthy to live", because, according to these judgments, they are "unproductive countrymen".'[41]

Bearing in mind that the British government proposed to have this sermon reprinted in pamphlet form and dropped all over Germany, one assumes that it must have been considered a fairly potent form of negative propaganda.

There was of course a huge difference between the notion of euthanasia espoused in Nazi Germany and that supported by the Voluntary Euthanasia Legalisation Society in Great Britain. The German programme had little to do with euthanasia in the sense of allowing the terminally ill the right to precipitate their own death prematurely. For this reason historians have usually presented the notions of euthanasia espoused in the respective countries as entirely separate.[42] In fact it has become common to see the term placed in quotation marks whenever reference is made to the Nazi programme.[43] Holocaust historian, Lucy Dawidowicz, has claimed that 'euthanasia' in the Nazi sense was not 'euthanasia' in our terms. Rather it was a 'codename' employed by the National Socialists as a euphemistic 'camouflage' for a murderous programme which involved the killing of 'various categories of persons because they were regarded as racially "valueless": deformed, insane, senile, or any combination thereof'.[44] While this view certainly has much to commend it, the fact that the same term was used ensured that the British euthanasia movement would not escape being tarred with the Nazi brush. Matters were not helped by the remarks of particular Nuremberg investigators. In a now famous article entitled 'Medical science under dictatorship',[45] American neurologist, Leo Alexander, argued that the colossal proportions which the Nazi programmes of extermination eventually assumed could be traced to 'small beginnings'. The beginning was a 'subtle shift' in the core beliefs of physicians, an acceptance of the view that there was such a concept as 'life not worthy to be lived'; a concept which was 'basic in the euthanasia movement'. While this attitude was concerned initially with cases of severe and chronic illness,

> Gradually the sphere of those to be included in this category was enlarged to encompass the socially unproductive, the ideologically unwanted, the racially unwanted and finally all non-Germans. But

it is important to realize that the infinitely small wedged-in lever from which this entire trend of mind received its impetus was the attitude toward the nonrehabilitable sick.[46]

Alexander's statement was perhaps the most explicit example of the thin-end-of-the-wedge, or slippery-slope argument, suggesting that the concept of worthless life was susceptible to progressive revision. The first step was an inherently dangerous one. Euthanasia of any description opened the way to escalating excesses.

This view dovetailed neatly with the arguments which had long been advanced by the opponents of euthanasia in Great Britain. These opponents realised extremely quickly that by associating these two very different notions of euthanasia with one another, the anti-euthanasia campaign was likely to prosper. The same tactic had been employed with comparative success in the period preceding the Bill of 1936 and clearly the revelations of the Nazi programme could be used to illustrate the apparent empirical truth of their arguments. Similarly, and understandably, the Voluntary Euthanasia Legalisation Society was anxious to dissociate itself from Nazi practices. As a result the narrative account of this period consists primarily of the struggle between these two opposing camps.

It should be made clear that this chapter does not claim that the British euthanasia movement harboured a clique of individuals intent on implementing Nazi style policies. As others have observed, there has 'been a lot of shoddy thinking and writing, making facile comparisons'.[47] Perhaps the most extreme example has been that of Bernard Schreiber who effectively asked whether Nazi medical crimes could have occurred elsewhere.[48] His argument was based on the supposition that the eugenics movement, the mental hygiene movement, and the movement in favour of euthanasia were all intimately related, and ultimately shared the same agenda in both Germany and Britain. He claimed that while particular movements sought ostensibly to introduce voluntary practices – notably voluntary sterilisation and voluntary euthanasia – this was a carefully considered diplomatic front, behind which lay the desire for more Draconian measures which were elements of an intolerant, eugenic ideology. In a German context, such claims had some empirical foundation, although even here Schreiber's claim over-simplifies the connections between the three movements. With regard to Great Britain, however, Schreiber's supposition is untenable. Relationships between these three movements certainly constituted one theme within the British euthanasia movement but the relationships need to be traced with precision, rather than with the broad brush of negative propaganda which Schreiber has wielded. The merit of Schreiber's account is that it questions those who have claimed that because the collective 'Volk' was regarded as an organism more important than its constituent parts, and that because of an alleged absence of a democratic tradition in early twentieth-century Germany the 'differences between these societies and our own minimise their usefulness in illuminating contemporary interest in euthanasia'.[49] It is suggested here that elements of the multifaceted rationale which informed the German euthanasia programme of 1939–45 were evident in Great Britain contemporaneously.

Seemingly aware of the damage which news of the Nazi programme could inflict upon the British euthanasia movement, Millard set about producing a pamphlet entitled *Merciful Release*[50] which stated explicitly that only voluntary euthanasia expressly requested by the sufferer was advocated by the Society. It explained that the Society's proposals did not extend to the application of euthanasia to 'imbeciles', 'mental defectives' or the 'hopelessly insane'. The objective was not to 'relieve the State of the burden of caring for the sick, mentally or physically, but to enable a sufferer who is already doomed to a painful death, humanly speaking, to anticipate that death if he so desires, by substituting a quick and painless death'.[51] These sentiments were reiterated in the Society's annual report of 1942. In fact, the report acknowledged that there were certain individuals who believed that euthanasia should be legalised for low-grade defectives. Proposals of this nature were predicated on the belief that life had nothing of substantive value to offer these poor 'human derelicts'.

Another motive for the prescribed destruction of such individuals was that it would ensure that there was no possibility of 'their reproducing their kind, and thus transmitting their terrible taint to future generations'. However, this survey of the British euthanasia movement has argued that this motive did not feature prominently among proposals for non-voluntary euthanasia in a British context. As we have often noted, the focus of most eugenists' concerns was the feeble-minded and it was among this class of mental defectives that fertility was considered to be most alarming and the dysgenic threat therefore greatest. Among the low-grade defectives, who

were often alleged to be scarcely human, the prospect of reproduc
tion was rather unlikely and the dysgenic consequences were
therefore negligible. As early as 1868 the eminent psychiatrist,
Henry Maudsley, had argued that the terminal point of degeneration was 'sterile idiocy'.[52] Among advocates of eugenic policies,
sterilisation for the feeble-minded persistently eclipsed notions of
eugenic euthanasia. It was only very rarely that the subjects of the
feeble-minded and euthanasia were mentioned in the same breath.
E. W. Barnes had done so on one occasion, but bearing in mind that
he spoke also of the 'sub-human' character of the recipients, it seems
likely that he was using the term 'feeble-minded' in a generic, catch-
all sense, rather than to refer to the sub-set of mental defect, i.e.
those closest to normal intelligence.

Economic considerations, however, were often cited in order to
justify the application of non-voluntary euthanasia to low-grade
defectives. As the Society's annual report suggested, advocates of
this proposal pointed to the 'needless burden which the maintenance of these unfortunates entails upon the community, diverting
resources which, they suggest could be better spent upon the
mentally normal'. Having conceded that such views were advanced
from time to time, the report made clear that these considerations
were entirely separate from those with which the Voluntary
Euthanasia Legalisation Society was concerned, 'for the underlying
principle of voluntary euthanasia is one of mercy and human justice
only'. In a clear attempt to extricate the British movement from all
association with Nazi excesses, it was stated that the Voluntary
Euthanasia Legalisation Society was not concerned with 'either
eugenics or national economics'.[53] But, as we have seen from the
remarks of numerous influential figures within the Society following the defeat of the Voluntary Euthanasia (Legalisation) Bill, this
was a rather sanitised appraisal of the views espoused within the
Society. Nevertheless, it was the first time that the Society had
published a document so free of ambiguity, and one might hypothesise that the revelations of the Nazi programme had forced the
Society to give serious consideration to these issues, as well as the
reality of proposals securing popular and parliamentary support.

In a speech entitled 'The legalisation of voluntary euthanasia',
Millard confronted the issue even more directly, when he stated
quite explicitly that the proposal of the Voluntary Euthanasia
Legalisation Society did not include the 'disposal of monsters or

deformed infants at birth or the euthanasia of the mentally deficient and the senile'. The focus of his speech was 'not euthanasia, but voluntary euthanasia'. Proposals for the legalised killing of such 'unfortunates' involved principles different to those pertaining to the case of voluntary euthanasia. Moreover, it was extremely doubtful whether a good case could be made for the application of 'euthanasia' to these 'non-responsible beings'. To grant a third party the right to determine when a particular life lacked the qualities which made life worthwhile, was a proposal which was viewed with great scepticism. The 'dangers of non-voluntary euthanasia' were 'exemplified by what the Nazi did'.[54] The Nazi programme had clearly made its mark.

However, prior to the publication of Shirer's articles, Millard had received a rather interesting letter from the Euthanasia Society of America. This Society had established very close links with the British organisation, modelling draft Bills on the Voluntary Euthanasia (Legalisation) Bill of 1936; Millard also served on its advisory council. In this letter one can identify clear sympathy with the notion of fusing eugenic ideology and ideas pertaining to euthanasia. While it is clearly inappropriate to ascribe such ideas to Millard merely through his association with the Society, the letter is worth noting as an example of the disparate reactions which revelations of the Nazi euthanasia programme aroused among advocates of euthanasia in the democratic societies of the western world. Referring to an article published in the *Herald Tribune* which had drawn attention to the administration of fatal doses of morphine and to the shooting of 'insane children' in German-occupied Poland, the letter remarked that the killing of such individuals was a 'great blessing' and it was merely unfortunate that it should have 'come about in this way'.[55]

The Voluntary Euthanasia Legalisation Society annual report of 1940 had been rather optimistic about the potential effects of war. It had suggested that 'ultimately and indirectly' the war was likely to 'influence' the cause beneficially. Pre-war views on a number of 'fundamental questions' were likely to undergo profound change as a consequence of the 'catastrophic upheaval' which accompanied war. A great deal that was 'old and out of date' would be 'burnt away leaving a fertile soil ready for the reception of much that is new'. It was considered likely that 'old established' ideas would tend to be supplanted by 'new ones' which may have been 'looked at askance in pre-war days'. Indeed, it suggested that there were already signs that changes of this variety were under way 'especially as regards certain important social questions which will gain ground through this tendency'.[56] Particular individuals evidently saw this new 'fertile soil' as the appropriate place to espouse ideas which were in many respects similar to those which drove the Nazi programme.

A letter to the Minister of Health from Miss E. Dyson in 1943 provides a particularly vivid example. Miss Dyson wished to draw attention to what she considered to be an 'important post-war' matter which impinged on the welfare of the country 'very much'. The subject was that of 'persons confined to Mental Homes, Institutions and Hospitals without hope of recovery'. It was suggested that from a human point of view the time had arrived at which individuals suffering from incurable mental and physical disease should be aided by a doctor to an early death. Miss Dyson claimed to speak from personal experience, as unfortunately in the last few months of her life, her mother 'went mental and had to go into a Mental Institution'. She suggested that it would have been far better for her mother's life to have been ended at the beginning of her infirmity than to have suffered in Hospital with her mind in 'chaos and not even knowing her own family'. Miss Dyson was also grieved by the sight of other sufferers such as 'a little child who would never be normal if she lived for years'.[57] Figures within the Voluntary Euthanasia Legalisation Society also espoused similar ideas.

During the period 1944–46 we find that little press attention was directed towards the issue of euthanasia. Bearing in mind that this was the time at which the full horrors of Nazi atrocities were being exposed, this is perhaps a little surprising. But the revelations from the East were concerned principally with the death camps used for the mass destruction of Jews, rather than the killing centres responsible for the disposal of the mentally defective. It seems reasonable to assume that the sheer numbers of Jews killed at Auschwitz and other camps meant that the euthanasia programme was rather lost sight of. Indeed, full documentation of the euthanasia programme occurred much later than that of the Final Solution which was accorded a much higher priority. It was perhaps for this reason that in the following years some individuals felt able to discuss the killing of mentally defective individuals.

At the annual conference of the co-operative movement in 1947, the Bishop of Birmingham, Dr E. W. Barnes, had spoken of a child born to 'apparently normal parents, pitiably defective in mind or body' and of the parents' sense of relief when the child dies. In such instances, Barnes was of the opinion that 'early euthanasia should be permitted under proper safeguards' and claimed that all present seemed to agree with his prescription of 'euthanasia for sub-human infants'.[58] For Barnes, opposition to the application of euthanasia in such cases was a consequence of 'sheer conservatism'.[59] Fighting off accusations that he had derived his proposals from Nazi practices, Barnes offered the defence that he had no knowledge of such activities: 'Euthanasia and sterilisation should be discussed without importing anti-Nazi prejudice.'[60] He claimed to have received several 'heartbreaking' letters from parents 'cursed' with a 'dreadfully sub-human' child, and suggested that visitors to hospitals where such children were looked after, must desire an alteration to the law. Despite his protestations, it is clear that Barnes had succeeded in fusing notions of euthanasia in the alleged interests of the individual concerned with the idea of purging society of eugenically and financially undesirable persons.

Barnes was something of a maverick and it must be acknowledged that Millard had been fairly successful in steering his Society in a conservative direction. His task had been aided somewhat by the deaths of such outspoken figures as C. J. Bond and Havelock Ellis. Nevertheless, once we begin to pursue the issue of euthanasia for defectives outside the confines of the Voluntary Euthanasia Legalisation Society we find that Barnes's sentiments were far from unique.

At the annual meeting of the Mental Hospitals' Association, at the Guildhall in London, attention was drawn to the alleged cowardice in dealing with the problem of low-grade mental defectives. Alderman Turner of Middlesbrough proposed that serious consideration should be given to euthanasia as a solution. He noted that there were 'children born into the world to-day who, we know from birth, are going to be of use neither to themselves nor to the nation. I say that it is a shame that they should be allowed to continue like that when you can do nothing for them'.[61] Once again we have an indication of how the value of human life could be assessed in terms of service to others, or to the nation as a whole. Making reference to Turner's speech, a letter to the *Yorkshire Post* remarked that 'this brutal statement indicates how far some have become infected with the principles of totalitarianism'.[62] While Turner may have been a marginal figure within the field of mental health, the case of A. F. Tredgold provides an example of a very prominent figure who shared similar ideas. As we have seen in previous chapters, Tredgold had written a classic work entitled *Mental Deficiency: Amentia*,[63] which was reprinted in several editions and served as the standard textbook for mental health. The edition of 1922 had noted that the problem of mental deficiency was a condition which had important, 'far-reaching' social and economic consequences. It had argued that in the interests of the 'defectives themselves' and of the 'general community' no 'civilised country' could afford to neglect the problem. The idea of a 'lethal chamber' was discussed and Tredgold suggested that in self-defence society would not necessarily be unjustified in employing such a method of 'ridding itself of its anti-social constituents'. Although arguments could be adduced both for and against this proposal, it was considered to be so 'clearly impracticable in the present state of public opinion', that it really required no further discussion. Tredgold stated plainly that '[w]e have to recognise that mental defectives exist, and must be allowed to exist, and the questions before us are as to the way in which the State can best deal with them, and the manner in which it can prevent their procreation.'[64] Having contemplated the extermination of mental defectives, Tredgold had swiftly rejected the idea, recognising that it was in any case unfeasible. He went on to outline remedial measures which included training and supervision, and methods for preventing the propagation of defectives including sterilisation, segregation and regulation of marriage, measures which might be termed typical eugenic solutions.

In 1947 the seventh edition of Tredgold's textbook was published and one might have supposed that his reservations about the extermination of defectives would have been cemented by the revelations of the Nazi euthanasia programme: his text suggests otherwise. The section on remedial measures now included a heading entitled 'Euthanasia'. It remarked that a suggestion had been made to the effect that the state should bring about the elimination of 'defectives and inefficient members within it'. Tredgold stated that the majority of people would logically agree that the absence of defectives would be beneficial. It was recognised, however, that many 'high-grade defectives' had a capacity for useful work and whatever view the state might adopt in the future, it was unlikely that public opinion would approve the destruction of such individuals at the present. With regard to the '80,000 or more idiots and imbeciles in the country' he believed the position to be very different. They were an economic dead-weight, incapable of profitable employment whose care in either institutions or homes absorbed considerable resources in terms of time, money and effort which could be 'utilized to better purpose'.

> [M]any of these defectives are utterly helpless, repulsive in appearance, and revolting in manners. Their existence is a perpetual source of worry and unhappiness to their parents, and those who live at home have a most disturbing influence upon other children and family life. With the present shortage of institutional accommodation there are thousands of mothers who are literally worn out in caring for these persons at home. In my opinion it would be an economical and humane procedure were their existence to be painlessly terminated, and I have no doubt, from personal experience, that this would be welcomed by a very large proportion of parents. It is doubtful if public opinion is yet ripe for this to be done compulsorily; but I am of the opinion that the time has come when euthanasia should be permitted at the request of a parent or guardian. It would clearly be necessary to devise adequate safeguards, but this would not present any practical difficulty.[65]

Such use of the term 'euthanasia' in the sense of the non-voluntary killing of the *non compos mentis*, replete with eugenic, economic and 'humanitarian' concerns is particularly striking. This combined with an intolerance for life which failed to fulfil minimum mental criteria and the revelations of the Nazi euthanasia programme appear to have led to an association in many people's minds between voluntary physician-assisted suicide and the wholesale slaughter of mental defectives. For the opponents of euthanasia these revelations seemed to confirm what they had suggested all along, namely that there was a slippery slope linking the two practices. Of course this is not to deny that the two practices are logically distinct from one another. As the *Church Times* recognised 'the agitation for legalising voluntary euthanasia ... may have suffered a set-back from the revelation by the Nazis of the dreadful lengths to which any approval of euthanasia may be carried' but, '[i]t can fairly be claimed ... that there is a great difference between recognising the power of the State to put its superfluous citizens to death and allowing individuals who are suffering from incurable and acutely painful diseases to arrange for the termination of their own lives'.[66] While the connection between the two concepts was thus not a logical one, the question remained whether it was an accurate descriptive one for the advocates of euthanasia in Great Britain. The article suggested that it was only the latter kind of euthanasia which had received support in Britain so far, but the question arose whether,

> once the principle underlying it is granted, there is any reasonable ground for stopping short at that point. Indeed, in 1935 the chairman of the Voluntary Euthanasia Legalisation Society made this statement at its inaugural meeting. 'As public opinion developed, and it became possible to form a truer estimate of the value of human life, further progress along preventive lines would be possible.'[67]

Others had clearly noted the inflationary remarks which we have observed throughout this study. While the Nazi euthanasia programme produced a marked conservatism on the part of Millard and the Voluntary Euthanasia Legalisation Society, who recognised the need to demarcate their proposals from the murderous policies of Nazi Germany, it is also clear that among others, such revelations seemed to instil new ideas, eliciting proposals which were more radical than ever.

In 1949 the *Evening Advertiser* carried the headline 'Should over 70s be killed off?'[68] Speaking on the 'The economist's view of euthanasia' at a meeting held by the Economics Society, a Mr D. S. Winton had claimed that if the birth rate was to persist at its present rate, the population in 1990 would be as low as 23 million, the number of old-age pensioners would have doubled, the relative working population would have halved, and thus the burden of supporting the older people would have quadrupled. While euthanasia was currently being considered as a release for those suffering unendurable pain, the changing age-structure of Great Britain suggested other applications. Winton enquired whether it would 'not be necessary in the future to consider it as a means of reducing the older section of the population'?[69] Of course this was a view advocated by the smallest of minorities, which found no expression within the Voluntary Euthanasia Legalisation Society, but it was in such remarkably poor taste that one wonders what kind of moral and ethical principles furnished the minds of many who were prepared to discuss the subject of euthanasia in a public forum.

Shortly after this example of crude fiscal reasoning had appeared, Dr Barnes was promptly back in the headlines. *The Times* and the *Daily Graphic* were among a host of papers which reported an extraordinary speech made at the Birmingham Rotary Club, at which Barnes spoke of overpopulation,[70] and suggested that the welfare state was likely to encourage an increase in the numbers of the 'slovenly', 'vicious', 'idle wasters of the community'. In proposing methods of reducing the population, Barnes made clear that the 'good-living', 'hard-working' should be preserved. But he also advocated euthanasia for obviously defective infants, and sterilisation of the unfit – which he defined as that 6 to 10 per cent of the population which is 'mentally below par' – as a means of 'promoting the social health of the community'.[71] Barnes's speech generated a deluge of readers' letters, a substantial number of which persisted in conflating eugenic, crude utilitarian, economic and allegedly humanitarian motivations in support of such proposals. A letter entitled 'Realistic view' endorsed the view that euthanasia and sterilisation should be employed to 'eliminate the degenerates, the feeble-minded, the parasites'. Such a policy was deemed to be both 'expedient' and 'rational' because these 'useless members' could only be a 'burden upon the economy'. Collectively these individuals were considered to be an 'exhausting factor in the life-blood of society'. Suggestions to the contrary were inspired simply by 'false sentiment'. The article argued that if the practice of euthanasia had been adopted twenty years ago, a great deal of 'ratepayers' money' could have been used to better effect. Under such circumstances it would have been unnecessary to devote resources to the upkeep of mental institutions 'where imbeciles could drag out useless lives'. In forthright language it was suggested that society should rid itself of 'the unfit, cut our fiscal cloth according to our economic coat, and England will be populated by Spartan men and women, able to plant the flag in any corner of the world'.[72]

It is extremely difficult to gauge the exact timbre of public opinion with regard to this matter, but while Dr Barnes claimed to have received considerable support from mothers of defective children, others took an entirely different view of humanitarianism, which extricated all reference to the worth of human life in terms of economic service to the community. Indeed, a letter published in the *Birmingham Evening Despatch*, provides a striking contrast to the sentiments expressed by Barnes. The letter was written by the mother of a 'backward' child who had died four years previously. Her daughter was incapable of walking, and doctors had indicated that the child would never be able to assimilate knowledge to 'any useful degree'. Despite these handicaps the child's death caused the 'light' to go out of her parents' lives. Dr Barnes's suggestion that 'backward babies should die for the good of the community' was rejected as a cruel and inhumane proposal.

> Let other nations, whose fate has been an object lesson to the world at large, out-Herod if they wish; but let us keep this country free from the taint of so-called racial superiority. Children, backward or otherwise are given to us for reasons no man can fathom. The 'backward' child may prove a blessing, and a 'normal' one has been known to be a curse. Strangely enough, the great majority of parents have more love and tenderness towards a handicapped child than to others not so afflicted. Patience and kindness can do much to improve such children. Anyone who knew my poor darling loved her, because of her sweet ways and pretty little face. Who is to say that such a one is not fit to live?[73]

While much of the debate during this period was heavily coloured by notions of non-voluntary euthanasia, discussion of voluntary euthanasia in its strictly limited form also took place. In many ways the debate continued to centre on the same issues which had divided the supporters and opponents of euthanasia ever since the 1870s. Particularly vociferous among the latter category during this period was the Catholic lobby, which launched a persistent assault upon the efforts to legalise euthanasia. Throughout the late 1940s, the Archbishop of Westminster, Cardinal Griffin championed the anti-euthanasia cause with a series of well-rehearsed arguments. Typical among these was the notion that a person's body is not his own property, but that of God. No one had the right to take his own life, or to permit others to take it for him. The curtailment of life was an area of Divine Prerogative.[74] The Pope had himself considered the question of euthanasia and vehemently opposed the practice, pointing to the 'false pity' which was used to 'condone immoral and fatal practices'. Suffering was considered to be a 'purifying' process and it was therefore inappropriate to deprive a human being of this by the means with which one concludes the life of an animal 'without reason and without immortality'.[75]

The retort of the Voluntary Euthanasia Legalisation Society was much as that advanced during the 1930s, and indeed from the 1870s onwards. Thus, we find recurrent reference to the 'hypocrisy' of the Roman Church, which, while trumpeting the doctrine of the sanctity of human life, failed to condemn the taking of life in numerous scenarios. In particular, it was noted that the Church of Rome, 'led by the Pope, blessed the Italian soldiers when setting out intent on the mass killing of the unfortunate Abyssinians, for this was legal killing, and therefore not murder. Most people, we think, would regard the Italo-Abyssinian war as a war of aggression if ever there was one'.[76]

In the course of 1949, the BBC transmitted a debate on euthanasia which provided the movement with considerable public exposure. Speaking in favour of voluntary euthanasia was Professor Major Greenwood, a member of the Society's Consultative Medical Council. Greenwood was opposed by an anonymous 'senior woman physician' and by Mr Richard O'Sullivan KC, a Roman Catholic barrister who based his opposition upon legal and religious grounds. He noted that euthanasia was a 'double felony', on the part of the recipient it was suicide and on the part of the physician it was murder. The 'tradition and office' of the law sought to protect life and not to facilitate its destruction. O'Sullivan could not imagine that people would be prepared to cast aside the 'tradition of ordinary English life and law and the Christian philosophy that inspires it in favour of a procedure that is alien to every right feeling in us'.[77]

There were, however, occasions when euthanasia at a more practical level intruded into the British press. In 1947 at the Voluntary Euthanasia Legalisation Society's annual meeting held in London, a member of the Society's Consultative Medical Council, Dr E. A. Barton, admitted to having practised euthanasia upon a patient who was dying in great pain and who expressly requested this form of relief. The most famous mercy-killing trial perhaps, took place in 1950, and ensured that for some time the question of euthanasia occupied the headlines. The trial took place in New Hampshire, USA, and the accused was Dr Herman Sander who was alleged to have killed a patient suffering from cancer. As the Society's annual report noted, the case had the effect of drawing 'public attention to the need for the legalisation of voluntary euthanasia more forcefully than anything else could have done'.[78] In the case notes of his terminally-ill patient, Sander had recorded the injection of 40 cc of air into the vein of his patient who died ten minutes later. Having been charged with murder, Sander was acquitted after his defence argued that the injection had been administered after the patient was in fact already dead. The Sander case generated a great deal of good publicity for the Voluntary Euthanasia Legalisation Society and served as something of an antidote to the torrent of negative propaganda which had furnished the preceding nine years. In fact the Society's annual report of 1949 claimed that 'very many must now realise as never before that there is a great reform to be brought about and a great injustice to be remedied'. In such circumstances the Society believed that an opportune moment was approaching at which their Bill could be re-introduced. This would be effected 'as soon as practicable'.[79]

The same year, the Society jointly with the Euthanasia Society of America was involved in petitioning the United Nations to include the right to voluntary euthanasia in its Declaration on Human Rights. It was unsuccessful, but it did manage to introduce a motion calling attention to the need for legislation on voluntary euthanasia to the House of Lords. In many respects the debate surrounding this motion was very similar to that of 1936. Arguments about humane practices, theological issues, and the ethics of physician-assisted suicide were all rehearsed in some detail. However, as we might have expected, far more attention was paid to the issue of euthanasia for the mentally defective, and the potential of the Voluntary Euthanasia (Legalisation) Bill for being extended at a subsequent stage. At various times, the notion of a slippery slope to euthanasia of the Nazi variety was raised. Once again the Society was not particularly fortunate in its selection of a peer to introduce the motion. Lord Chorley suggested that one objection to the Bill might be that it did not go far enough, 'because it applies only to adults and does not apply to children who come into the world deaf, dumb and crippled, and who have a much better case than those for whom the Bill provides'.[80] In an almost identical fashion to Lord Ponsonby in 1936, in revealing the way in which the Bill might be expanded, Lord Chorley had handed the opposition all the requisite ammunition with which to fire home their point. Indeed, he went on to note, 'That may be so, but we must go step by step.'[81]

While admittedly suggesting that what the Society had in mind was only that a 'person who is able to come to a decision for himself who should be granted this method of leaving his life'[82] the ambiguity had been noted. Referring to Chorley's *faux pas* the Archbishop of York remarked that '[i]f once we begin to allow legislation of this kind we put our feet on a very slippery slope.'[83] Clearly with the Nazi Euthanasia programme in mind, the Archbishop raised a rhetorical question: if this right was to be granted in 'connection with excessive pain', why should it not also be granted to those who are born feeble-minded? And to those who are so severely crippled that they are of 'no service to the nation', why should such a measure not be applied to the occupants of the nation's mental asylums? The Archbishop observed that Germany had 'placed its feet on this slippery slope'. The euthanasia programme had had small beginnings but during the war had transformed into a large-scale operation which was responsible for the destruction of large numbers of people who were considered 'useless mouths in a time of emergency'. He was of the opinion that to start legislating on this issue was a 'real danger' which would seriously undermine the value attached to human life.[84]

Arguments of the von Galen variety were difficult to dislodge despite the protestations of Lord Chorley that his Society was concerned only with voluntary euthanasia. Precisely the same concerns were raised by Lord Amulree,[85] and by the Lord Chancellor, Viscount Jowitt.[86] Speaking as a doctor, Lord Haden-Guest also found the whole issue more than a little disconcerting. Turning to the issue of euthanasia for mentally defective children, he embarked upon a forceful denunciation of the practice, in which he drew attention to the pernicious reasoning which seemed to motivate particular advocates of euthanasia. Having visited an institution for extreme cases of physical and mental defect, he had seen children that were small often confined to a bed or crib with 'tiny little heads ... animal-like' in appearance. Noting that these children were incurable, Haden-Guest raised the rhetorical question of why these children should not be included in the proposed euthanasia reforms. Such individuals absorbed the time and energy of doctors and nurses and thereby consumed the finances of the general public. The idea of extending the practice to 'hopeless lunatics' was also noted. With a cutting outburst, Haden-Guest enquired why society should not go the 'whole "Hitler hog" and set up concentration camps to which we could send the people whom we do not like, on the ground that they are mentally and medically unfit?' He concluded by noting that it was the duty of the medical

profession to cure and not 'to go into this pathological excursion
into the realms of the unconscious and bring out of it some horrible
idea of euthanasia for certain classes of people'.[87] Such was the
overwhelming opposition to the proposals advanced by Lord
Chorley, that he withdrew his motion without forcing a division of
the House.

The following year C. P. Blacker, the General Secretary of the
Eugenics Society delivered a speech to the members of the Eugenics
Society, with the title '"Eugenic" experiments conducted by the
Nazi on human subjects.'[88] This speech was a thinly veiled attempt
to disassociate the British eugenics movement from the 'eugenic'
practices which took place during the Third Reich. Noting that
Galton had declared eugenics to be a 'merciful creed', Blacker
suggested that it was therefore 'unjust and deplorable that the word
eugenics should be connected with Nazi racialist practices. But
unfortunately the connection has been established in the minds of
many people.'[89] Bearing in mind that advocates of eugenic euthanasia often claimed that the practice was a merciful one which ended
the hellish existence of mentally incompetent sub-humans,
Blacker's statement was not entirely reassuring. He remarked that
whatever view one held with regard to the Nazi policies of sterilisation 'which was in part made public' and the covert euthanasia
programme, documentary evidence seemed to indicate that these
policies were executed with a 'certain discrimination' initially at
least. In theory individuals could appeal to a 'higher eugenic court'
in order to dispute the validity of compulsory sterilisation orders.
With regard to the euthanasia programme, Blacker noted that 'the
incurably insane person was sent for a period of one to three
months to an observation centre before being sent elsewhere to be
liquidated, and for the most part these people were mercifully
killed'.[90]

Blacker's primary concern seemed to be that two years into the
war, these programmes began to operate more arbitrarily. There
seemed to be little disagreement with the underlying principles.
Evidently, Blacker did not regard all human life as equally valuable.
Blacker considered that 'on a scale of turpitude' the application of
euthanasia to individuals suffering from insanity 'ranked lower'
than human vivisection. He suggested that if one rejected the
account of mass starvation to which 'one doctor' had alluded,[91]
'these people were mercifully killed'. Blacker proceeded to note that

the 'idea of merciful killing' was not unknown in Great Britain where a Society sought to promote it on a voluntary basis, for people suffering from incurable and painful illnesses.[92] If figures of Blacker's calibre were prepared to discuss the Nazi euthanasia programme and the Voluntary Euthanasia Legalisation Society in the same breath it was hardly surprising that the slippery-slope argument was so prevalent throughout this period.

This chapter has sought to highlight the plurality of reactions which the revelations of the Nazi euthanasia programme elicited among the participants of the euthanasia debate in Great Britain. In general this period was marked by the parallel efforts of the Voluntary Euthanasia Legalisation Society to distance itself from notions of compulsory euthanasia for the mentally defective and the anti-euthanasiasts' attempts to conflate voluntary and non-voluntary euthanasia. The true originality of this chapter, however, lies in its exposure of the rich discussion concerning non-voluntary euthanasia for defectives which took place after 1941. As noted throughout the book, such discussion deserves a far more central place in the history of the British euthanasia movement than it has received hitherto. After 1941 the intimate association which was established between the term 'euthanasia' and the Nazi practice of non-voluntary killing for defectives helped to obstruct legislative reform until well into the second half of the twentieth century. While it is clear that many individuals were repelled by the revelations of the Nazi euthanasia programme, it is also clear that others were not so perturbed. Indeed the frequency of proposals for non-voluntary euthanasia tended to increase in this period. Such sentiment saddled the British euthanasia movement with profound problems.

Notes

1   CMAC/SA/VES/A.11/1 Voluntary Euthanasia Legalisation Society First Annual Report and Statement of Accounts, Presented at the Annual Meeting held in London, 25 Feb. 1937, p. 11.
2   *Ibid.*, p. 7.
3   CMAC/SA/VES/A.11/14 Annual Report (AR) for the year ending 31 Dec. 1950, p. 4.
4   *Journal of the American Medical Association*, 1950, Vol. 143, Organization Section, p. 561.
5   *BMJ*, 1969, Vol. 2, supplement, p. 41.
6   The most comprehensive English language accounts of the Nazi euthanasia

programme are: Michael Burleigh, *Death and Deliverance: 'Euthanasia' in Germany 1900–45* (Cambridge, 1993); Henry Friedlander, *The Origins of Nazi Genocide: From Euthanasia to the Final Solution* (Chapel Hill, 1995).

7   I. Van der Sluis, 'The movement for euthanasia 1875–1975', *Janus*, Vol. 66, p. 160.

8   Mathew Thomson, *The Problem of Mental Deficiency: Eugenics, Democracy, and Social Policy in Britain c. 1870–1959* (Oxford, 1998).

9   *Ibid.*, p. 279.

10 *Ibid.*, p. 284.

11 CMAC/SA/VES/B.6 Extract from an address to the University of Oxford, *Manchester Guardian*, 8 Mar. 1937.

12 CMAC/SA/VES/B.6 *Manchester Guardian*, 8 Mar. 1937.

13 See, John Barnes, *Ahead of his Age: Bishop Barnes of Birmingham* (London, 1979) pp. 425–6.

14 CMAC/SA/VES/B.6 *Leicester Evening Mail*, 13 Nov. 1937.

15 CMAC/SA/VES/B.6 *Daily Sketch*, 26 Mar. 1938.

16 CMAC/SA/VES/B.6 *Daily Express*, 26 Mar. 1938.

17 CMAC/SA/VES/B.6 *Daily Sketch*, 30 Mar. 1938.

18 *Ibid.*

19 CMAC/SA/VES/A.11/3 AR for the year ending 31 Dec. 1938.

20 CMAC/SA/VES/A.11/4 AR for the year ending 31 Dec. 1939, p.4.

21 CMAC/SA/VES/A.11/5 AR for the year ending 31 Dec. 1940.

22 CMAC/SA/VES/A.11/6 AR for the year ending 31 Dec. 1941.

23 CMAC/SA/VES/A.11/4 AR for the year ending 31 Dec. 1939, p. 5.

24 *Ibid.*, p. 6.

25 Public Record Office (PRO) PRO/FO 37124392 1940 Reported destruction of mentally defective and infirm persons: (C12096/C12816/C1375616/18); PRO/FO 37126526 (C1130/21/18), 26518 (C2874/19/18), 26534 (C231/191/18), 26508 (C60/18/18; C443/18/18), 26509 (C3214/18/18), 26510 (C5379/18/18; C4789/18/18), 26513 (C11451/18/18; C10965/18/18; C11335/18/18) 1941 Reported killing of aged, infirm and insane persons and abnormal children, and seriously maimed casualties: possible utilisation for experiments on effect of poison gas: suggested utilisation for British whispering campaign.

26 CMAC/SA/VES/B.6 Extract from the 'Acta Apostolicae Sedis', 16 Dec. 1940, Ser. II, v. VII. Num. 13, cited in the *Daily Mirror*, 21 May 1941.

27 *Ibid.*

28 CMAC/SA/VES/B.6 *Daily Mirror*, 21 May 1941.

29 CMAC/SA/VES/B.6 Letter from Helena M. Wakerly, *Leicester Mercury*, 30 May 1941.

30 CMAC/SA/VES/B.6 *Daily Mirror*, 21 May 1941.

31 *Ibid.*

32 *Ibid.*

33 See I. Van der Sluis, 'The movement for euthanasia', pp. 173–92 ; Burleigh, *Death and Deliverance*, pp. 11–42.

34 Gerkan's Bill is reproduced in Burleigh, *Death and Deliverance*, pp. 13–14.

35 Adolf Hitler, *Mein Kampf*, with introduction by D. C. Watt, p. 259.

36 J. Noakes and G. Pridham (eds), *Nazism 1919–1945, vol. 3: Foreign Policy, War and Racial Extermination* (Exeter, 1988) p. 1002.

37 Paul Weindling, *Health, Race and German Politics Between National Unification and Nazism, 1870–1945* (Cambridge, 1989) p. 578.

38 Friedlander, *Origins of Nazi Genocide*, pp. 39–40. This interpretation has recently been modified by the work of Benzenhöfer which suggests that while there was a child 'K' born with some defect, the child was born later than previously thought. The case was used as a retrospective legitimisation for the 'Euthanasia' programme. See U. Bezenhöfer, 'Kindereuthanasie im *Dritten Reich*, Der Fall "Kind Knauer"', *Deutsches Ärteblatt*, 95, Heft, 8 Mai 1998, pp. 954–5.

39 W. G. Lennox, 'Should they live? Certain economic aspects of medicine,' American Scholar, 7 (1938) pp. 454–66; Foster Kennedy, 'The problem of social control of the congenitally defective: education, sterilisation, euthanasia,' *American Journal of Psychiatry*, 99 (1942) pp. 13–16; Alexis Carrel, *Man the Unknown* (London, 1936) p. 296; Maureen Gildea, *Euthanasia: A Review of the American Literature*, senior thesis, Harvard University, 1983.

40 Friedlander, *Origins of Nazi Genocide*, pp. 80–1.

41 CMAC/SA/VES/B.6 Count von Galen extract cited in the *Sunday Chronicle*, 10 Nov. 1941.

42 Ezekiel Emanuel, 'The history of euthanasia debates in the United States and Britain', *Annals of Internal Medicine*, Vol. 121, No. 10, pp. 793–802.

43 See for example Michael Burleigh, *Death and Deliverance*.

44 *The Hastings Center Report*, Vol. 6, No. 4, Aug. 1976, p. 3.

45 Leo Alexander, 'Medical science under dictatorship', *New England Journal of Medicine*, Vol. 241, No. 2, 14 Jul. 1949, pp. 39–47.

46 *Ibid.*, p.44.

47 *Hastings Center Report*, Vol. 6, No. 4, Aug. 1976, p. 4.

48 Bernard Schreiber, *The Men Behind Hitler* (London, 1972).

49 Emanuel, 'The history of euthanasia debates', p. 793.

50 CMAC/SA/VES/C.3 Dr C. Killick Millard, *Merciful Release*, 31 Oct. 1941.

51 *Ibid.*

52 Henry Maudsley, *The Physiology and Pathology of Mind* (London, 1868) pp. 246–7.

53 CMAC/SA/VES/A.11/7 AR for the year ending 31 Dec. 1942.

54 CMAC/SA/VES/C.4 *The Legalisation of Voluntary Euthanasia*, A speech for delivery by Killick Millard c. 1941.

55 CMAC/SA/VES/A.20 Correspondence from the Euthanasia Society of America to Dr C. Killick Millard, from Mrs R. L. Mitchell, Secretary, 7 May 1940.

56 CMAC/SA/VES/A.11/7 AR for the year ending 31 Dec. 1942.

57 PRO/MH58/650 Letter to the Minister of Health from Miss E. Dyson, 14 July 1943.

58 CMAC/SA/VES/B.6 Letter to the Editor from E. W. Birmingham, *Manchester Guardian*, 17 May 1947.

59 *Ibid.*

60 *Ibid.*

61 CMAC/SA/VES/B.6 The source and date of this extract are uncertain, but surrounding documents suggest that it is probably from the *Yorkshire Post c.* 16 July 1947.

62 CMAC/SA/VES/B.6 Letter from J. M. Cameron, *Yorkshire Post*, 26 July 1947.

63 A. F. Tredgold, *Mental Deficiency: Amentia* (London, 1908).

64 Tredgold, *Mental Deficiency: Amentia*, 3rd edn (London, 1922) pp. 532–3.

65 Tredgold, *Mental Deficiency: Amentia*, 7th edn (London, 1947) p. 491.

66 CMAC/SA/VES/B.7 *The Church Times*, 7 Nov. 1947.
67 *Ibid.*
68 CMAC/SA/VES/B.7 *Evening Advertiser*, 25 Mar. 1949.
69 *Ibid.*
70 John Barnes, *Ahead of his Age: Bishop Barnes of Birmingham* (London, 1979) p. 425.
71 CMAC/SA/VES/B.7 *Yorkshire Post*, 29 Nov. 1949.
72 CMAC/SA/VES/B.7 Reader's letter, *Birmingham Evening Despatch*, 1 Dec. 1949.
73 CMAC/SA/VES/B.7 *Birmingham Evening Despatch*, 30 Nov. 1949.
74 *Catholic Times*, 10 Oct. 1947.
75 Cited in *The Universe*, 19 Sep. 1947.
76 CMAC/SA/VES/A.11/11 AR for the year ending 3 Dec. 1947.
77 *Ibid.*
78 CMAC/SA/VES/A.11/11 AR for the year ending 31 Dec. 1947.
79 CMAC/SA/VES/A.11/13 AR for the year ending 31 Dec. 1949.
80 *House of Lords Debate (H.L. Deb.)* 28 Nov. 1950, c. 559.
81 *Ibid.*
82 *Ibid.*
83 *Ibid.*, c. 563.
84 *Ibid.*, c. 564.
85 *Ibid.*, c. 577.
86 *Ibid.*, c. 595.
87 *Ibid.*, c. 583.
88 Blacker had been invited to examine material relating to eugenics to see if it had any scientific value, as part of Lord Moran's Commission, which was established to investigate the war crimes of German doctors.
89 Blacker Papers, Wellcome Unit for the History of Medicine, Oxford (BL) BL/18.3.27 '"Eugenic" experiments conducted by the Nazis on human subjects', by C. P. Blacker. Paper given to a Members' Meeting of the Society on 14 Dec. 1951, p. 10.
90 *Ibid.*, p. 12.
91 This practice was in fact genuine, see Burleigh, *Death and Deliverance*, p. 46.
92 Blacker, '"Eugenic" experiments', p. 17.

6

The 1950s: a difficult decade

The House of Lords debate on 28 November 1950 had been an igno-
minious failure for the supporters of voluntary euthanasia. So
overwhelming was the opposition that Lord Chorley withdrew his
motion without forcing a division of the House. With considerable
regret Charles Killick Millard had to acknowledge that all five
medical peers had spoken against Chorley's motion.[1] In the same
year the World Medical Association and the British Medical
Association both issued unambiguous statements condemning the
practice of euthanasia.[2] The persistent problems which the euthanasia movement had encountered in securing official support from the
organs of the medical profession were thus reinforced. By the early
1950s the prospects for legislative reform seemed less propitious
than at any time since the foundation of the Voluntary Euthanasia
Legalisation Society in 1935. Euthanasia had always been politically
a marginal issue and in the post-war environment of reconstruction
and the welfare state mercy-killing was not particularly pressing. It
suffered, too, by association with the Nazi practice of putting to
death mental and physical defectives. Nor was the moral climate of
the 1950s especially conducive to reform; moralistic legislation then
being conspicuous by its absence.

There were also a number of more straightforward pragmatic
reasons which hindered progress through much of the 1950s. These
factors included an effective opposition, an ageing membership,
loss of leadership and developments in palliative care. Not until the
end of the decade did advances in medical technology show signs
of changing this picture. These developments served to complicate
considerably medico-ethical issues and in so doing made the question of euthanasia more pertinent than it had been hitherto.

Politically and in other ways the 1950s were a conservative

decade. In this light the Euthanasia Society's distinct lack of progress is perhaps not overly surprising. But it was not the only cause which suffered. Parliamentary attempts to legalise abortion were thwarted on two separate occasions and the Abortion Law Reform Association seemed to be at something of a low ebb.[3] The policing of homosexuality was firm[4] and there was no legislative reform of the much-criticised divorce law or death penalty. Yet euthanasia was a reform cause which seems to have encountered special difficulty, for whereas all these causes made some progress in the 1950s and triumphed in the 1960s, euthanasia did not. The depiction of 1960s as a permissive era during which attitudes towards sexuality and moral issues more broadly were revolutionised[5] should be qualified with reference to important developments occurring in the 1950s which served as the prerequisites for the more tangible legislative reforms of the following decade.[6]

During the 1950s, for example, the medical profession was beginning to offer cautious support for the idea of abortion law reform, particularly where there was the possibility of the birth of a defective infant.[7] The idea was also gaining ground in 'the community at large'.[8] With regard to homosexual law reform, Leo Abse's Sexual Offences Act of 1967 would have been inconceivable without the appointment and progressive conclusions of the Wolfenden Committee.[9] The punitive approach towards homosexuality had also prompted calls for its legalisation from *The Times*.[10] Similarly, although it was not until 1969 that the Divorce Law was reformed debate about matrimonial causes was in full swing.[11] In all these areas there was a strong, vocal and tangible case for legislative reform. Illegal abortion was a principal cause of maternal deaths and although there was some uncertainty, abortion on therapeutic grounds was probably already legal. Divorce had also increased inexorably.[12] Euthanasia, on the other hand, was less visible. Prosecutions almost never occurred, and when they did, they usually concerned family members who had killed relatives who were either dying or mentally defective. In Britain no physician had ever been prosecuted for administering a fatal dose of narcotics to a patient who was terminally ill. The law seemed to be fairly flexible and did not eye too closely the actions of the physician at the deathbed. In contrast to the abortion movement, the supporters of euthanasia had persistently failed to secure the backing of the

British Medical Association. In tandem with numerous arguments against euthanasia this had made legislative reform particularly problematic.

Throughout the early 1950s scaremongering tactics initiated by Catholic opponents of euthanasia received considerable press coverage. Most notable among these were the claims of Dr Halliday Sutherland to the effect that doctors in England frequently administered euthanasia to patients whom they regarded as nuisances.[13] Intermittent references to Nazi practices also served to taint the notion of voluntary euthanasia with images of non-voluntary killing.[14] The most important factors in stifling the advance of the euthanasia movement, however, were the important changes in personnel brought about by the resignations and deaths of key figures within the Society.

As an interest group concerned with the relief of suffering in terminal illnesses it is hardly surprising that the Voluntary Euthanasia Legalisation Society should attract old people. Millard and Bond had both pioneered the campaign comparatively late in life and the majority of the Society's members were senior citizens. Lord Moynihan, the first President of the Society, had died at the age of seventy-one shortly before the Voluntary Euthanasia (Legalisation) Bill of 1936 was introduced to the House of Lords. Nor was it overly surprising that in the wake of the Lords' defeat the seventy-seven-year-old Lord Denman should tender his resignation, having held the position of President since 1946, citing his 'advancing years' as the cause.[15] Although the position of President was undoubtedly of considerable importance within the Society it was the Honorary Secretary, Charles Killick Millard, who was the linchpin of the euthanasia movement. A man of seemingly inexhaustible energy Millard had devoted tremendous effort and enthusiasm to the campaign. It was thus with great sadness that in the course of 1951 he resigned from the Society because of defective circulation which had left him bedridden. On 7 March 1952 shortly after dictating the annual report for 1951 Millard died leaving an already struggling Society bereft of inspiration and direction. The following year the outspoken Bishop of Birmingham, Dr E. W. Barnes, died at the age of seventy-nine.[16] The euthanasia movement had been deprived of two enormously charismatic figures capable of generating a great deal of publicity. The weakness of the Society's leadership was compounded in 1953 when Dr N. I. Spriggs announced that he was becoming 'increasingly old and lame' and was looking forward to the time when he could pass on the chairmanship, which he had accepted on only a temporary basis as a favour to Millard, to a younger man.[17] The seventy-seven-year-old Canon F. R. C. Payne, a member of the original executive committee, also tendered his resignation.

With no natural successor the Society began looking for a new Honorary Secretary. An important qualification was that the candidate should live in or near London. Millard had been keen for the organisation to find a London headquarters, close to the locus of power. Since its inception the Society had been based in Leicester, where most of the Committee resided, but it was recognised that this was a rather parochial base, which prevented the Society from being truly influential. The appointment of Mr R. S. W. Pollard, a London solicitor, to the position of Honorary Secretary in 1954 thus realised 'one of the strongest hopes of the Founder and first Honorary Secretary of the Society ... who appreciated the advantages to educational work, propaganda and political agitation resulting from an office in the capital'.[18] The relocation of the Society was only one indication of comprehensive changes which were in the pipeline.

Having assumed the position of Honorary Secretary, Pollard urged the members to play a more active role in securing legislative reform, remarking that 'if in the future, the committee asked members to take any action, they would respond and that by facing the difficulties together, the Society would eventually triumph'.[19] This marked an important shift in approach which was set out in Pollard's memorandum 'Development and Future Policy of the Society' presented at a meeting of the Executive Committee held in October 1954. This document sought to establish an agenda for the way in which the Society should be developed and the role which members could be expected to play. In broad terms it called on members to become more active, whereas hitherto a small number of members, notably the Executive Committee, had undertaken the majority of work, while ordinary members merely pledged their moral support.

Perhaps the most notable shift was towards a more populist approach. Support from the 'middle and upper classes' constituted the bulwark of the movement. Among the 'thinking and more intelligent members of the community' there was considerable support but elsewhere the movement was practically unknown, particularly among the 'working class'. This was chiefly because the Society had 'deliberately concentrated' its propaganda towards the upper echelons of society, a fact borne out by the composition of its 'list of distinguished supporters'.[20] This was of course a reasonably effective tool of propaganda in its own right which continued to serve a useful purpose. But while the Society had relied on writing to people listed in the pages of *Who's Who*, a small proportion of whom replied, it was recognised that in the future more effort would need to be made with a wider public. Not only was this important from the perspective of spreading the word it was also necessary from a financial point of view. Previously the Society had relied upon a one-off fee from members, but with expenditure outstripping income it was necessary to request an annual fee and seek new members if the Society's precarious finances were to be restored. Matters were not helped by an elderly membership afflicted with a high level of natural 'wastage'. The membership records of the Society also needed to be put in some sort of order. Of particular importance was the need to prune the unwieldy 'paper' membership down to a 'list of real paying and supporting members'. To this effect the membership list was reduced from 1,500 members to 1,060 in the course of 1955, a mere 226 of whom had been recorded as 'paying or life members'.[21]

Identifying the problem was of course substantially easier than solving it. The question of how a broader membership could be attracted was extremely difficult. In its infancy the Society had received a great deal of media attention because of its novelty value but by the 1950s the subject seemed to be considerably less newsworthy. 'Except as part of a campaign by the Society' national newspapers usually published letters only if they 'related to some current case or topic'.[22]

Editors of local newspapers, however, were slightly more receptive to readers' letters and here the members could be expected to play a more active role. Indeed it was hoped that much progress could be made at the local level. It was felt that efforts should be made to introduce the topic of euthanasia to local debating societies and other associations. Rotary Clubs, Townswomen's Guilds, Women's Co-operative Guilds, Ethical Societies, and the Professional Association of Women's Clubs were all identified as potential arenas for discussion. The Society could offer to provide speakers for these meetings, but as the Honorary Secretary could only fulfil a handful of engagements, it would be necessary to establish a panel of speakers and prepare speakers' notes.[23] Ordinary members could initiate meetings, write letters to the local press, supply literature to their friends, but could also play a more explicitly political role. At the time of general elections it was recommended that members should approach candidates from all parties to make clear their views on euthanasia. Such a policy might help to convince potential MPs that there was a demand for euthanasia which deserved some consideration. It was acknowledged, however, that approaches of this nature could do little more. A euthanasia lobby could never be electorally influential and it was naive to suppose that a prospective Member of Parliament would include a strong stance on euthanasia as part of his manifesto. Few votes were to be won by taking a strong stance on a highly controversial issue which held little political currency. Indeed, Pollard acknowledged that it was 'useless for the Society to write direct to candidates'; approach through a constituent was eminently preferable. Even more important was 'the need for members to raise the problem with their existing local Members of Parliament and to interest them in the question'.[24] This seems to have been a partial admission that the earlier policy of attempting to secure legislative reform by networking with influential political players had not been very successful.

A switch towards grass-roots pressure was now being advocated as an alternative line of attack. When progress had been made on this front the Society could attempt to bring about a euthanasia debate in the House of Commons 'either on a private member's bill or on a general motion for the reform of the law'.[25] Prior to this date efforts to introduce legislative reform had always been concentrated on the House of Lords; an approach which seems to have had considerable logic. Electorally unaccountable, the Lords was the ideal environment for discussing contentious issues. Several members of the House were also distinguished professionals from the fields of medicine and law who would be required to demonstrate the existence of professional support from their respective spheres if legislative reform were to take place. However, over the course of twenty years these distinguished individuals had not been able to effect the desired reform. Elite networking had not been successful. The membership was now asked to become more involved. This was a logical step if only for the reason that Millard had carried an enormous workload which no one else could or would be prepared to assume. The Society was also anxious that an increasingly politicised working class should be targeted. In this sense it was perhaps understandable that the efforts to legalise voluntary euthanasia should aim at the House of Commons.

In Pollard's view there were three stages necessary in every reform. The first stage was to 'waken people from apathy, indifference and ignorance'. This was to be followed by a phase of debate when the proponents of a particular policy would be required to engage in 'controversy, often with unscrupulous opponents'. The third and final stage would be the 'overcoming of the opposition and victory'.[26] In Pollard's opinion the Society remained firmly rooted between stages one and two. Before the matter could be brought before Parliament again it would be necessary to effect 'a great deal more public education and the demand for voluntary euthanasia must also be made more widespread and vocal'.[27] This was in effect a frank admission that the Society had not made much progress.

Having changed the composition of the Executive Committee, prepared a set of speakers' notes, and established a panel of speakers – albeit weak in number – the euthanasia movement still found its task decidedly hard going. The publicity which the Society managed to generate for itself was not only low-key it was also less than plentiful. In the course of 1955 the Society had addressed meetings of 'the New Generation Group attached to the Hampstead Ethical Society, a Rotary luncheon meeting in Essex, and … the Christchurch Debating Society' which defeated a motion in favour of legalising voluntary euthanasia. The annual report said it was difficult to organise meetings where euthanasia could be discussed. It had become increasingly apparent that the only way to organise meetings on the subject was 'by personal contact and suggestion'. During the year the Society had approached Rotary Clubs, Townswomen's Guilds, the Socialist Medical Association and the British Medical Association, but the response had been 'disappointing'. Most of these organisations were not even prepared to tell their members that speakers were available, and when they had, the 'request for speakers was small'. In 1935, by contrast, the British Medical Association had provided Tavistock House free of charge to the Voluntary Euthanasia Legalisation Society for the purposes of a debate even though it did not approve of euthanasia. Not only had the Society moved towards more low-key meetings, it was failing even on this front. In fact there was nothing new about discussing euthanasia at local society meetings, as this had been a central part of the Voluntary Euthanasia Legalisation Society's approach throughout the 1930s and 1940s. Indeed, the approach adopted in the early 1950s was to some extent a scaling down rather than a reasoned and deliberate shift.

Alongside the change of personnel, the annual general meeting of 1955 voted to change the name of the Society to the Euthanasia Society. Although technically correct, the 'Voluntary Euthanasia Legalisation Society' was thought by 'many to be cumbersome and in practice, the Society was generally known as VELS. It was difficult to find the name in the telephone directory and enquiries could easily be discouraged.'[28] Appended to the new name was the sub-title 'A Society for obtaining the legalisation of Voluntary Euthanasia'. It seems that this had been included to prevent the misapprehension that the objectives of the Society had moved towards a more expansive notion of euthanasia. Nevertheless, bearing in mind the Society's persistent difficulty in convincing opponents that its proposals were moderate – evidenced most recently by the 1950 House of Lords' debate – the name change was perhaps not the most politic gesture.

Although there was a pronounced scarcity of press articles on euthanasia during this period, euthanasia for the *non compos mentis* was one of the few subjects which could generate attention. In 1955, for example, *The Times* carried a headline reporting the proposal of 'Euthanasia of babies in certain cases'[29] made by Alderman W. L. Dingley, chairman of the Mental Health Committee of the Association of Hospital Management Committee, while giving evidence before the Royal Commission on the Law Relating to Mental Illness and Mental Deficiency. Dingley had suggested that the parents of 'physically and mentally abnormal children' should be able to consent to euthanasia if there was not the 'slightest hope' for the child.[30] He repeated his views on the subject later in the year at the first convention of the newly incorporated National Society for Mentally Handicapped Children.[31] Proposals of this nature were something of an embarrassment for a society which ostensibly advocated only voluntary euthanasia for the *compos mentis*. But, as we will note at numerous points throughout this chapter, discussion of euthanasia for defectives continued to accompany discussion of voluntary euthanasia. Indeed, towards the end of the 1950s the question of euthanasia for severely handicapped infants became even more frequent.

After changing its name, issuing such a comprehensive reappraisal of its tactics and making many proposals for realignment, the resignation of Mr Pollard due to increased pressure of business in 1956 came as a severe blow to the Society. The captain had abandoned a ship which was keeping afloat only with difficulties. In the interim Miss G. F. Fishwick assumed the title Honorary Secretary but shared the workload with the Society's assistant secretary Miss Audrey Jupp. In the wake of Pollard's resignation Charles Killick Millard's son, Maurice, remarked that he had 'come to the scene, taken the society up and breathed new life into it'. It was certainly true that he had taken over the leadership while the Society was at its lowest ebb, but it was less clear that Pollard had played the resuscitatory role which Maurice Millard politely suggested. Indeed, Pollard had noted himself that it was becoming increasingly apparent that 'no immediate change in the law' could be looked for. In the same year the last remaining member of the original Executive Committee, Revd A. S. Hurn, announced his resignation along with that of three other members of the Executive Committee. Maurice Millard also resigned from the position of Chairman and was replaced by Dr C. K. MacDonald, giving the Society an almost entirely new leadership.

The Society's lack of progress prompted the launch of its most comprehensive and vigorous publicity campaign. In the course of 1957 advertisements were posted in the London Underground. For the first thirteen weeks these posters bore a large question mark with a caption reading 'What is euthanasia?' followed by the name and address of the Society. During the following thirteen weeks a second poster was used which read 'The Euthanasia Society believes that incurable sufferers should have the right to choose a Merciful Death.'[32] These posters were hardly the most inspired or eye-catching, but the wording of the Society's posters had to take the form of a question in order to comply with the conditions laid down by the 'authorities'. Any wording which might be considered 'controversial' was deemed unacceptable. This form of advertising was enlarged the following year. Posters were placed in British Electric trains on the Southern section. It was also decided to take

THE
EUTHANASIA SOCIETY
BELIEVES

that incurable sufferers
should have the right to
choose a Merciful Death

The Euthanasia Society

13 PRINCE OF WALES TERRACE
LONDON, W.8

Telephone: WEstern 7770

WHAT IS
EUTHANASIA

?

Write to

The Euthanasia Society

13 PRINCE OF WALES TERRACE
LONDON, W.8

Telephone: WEstern 7770

2 and 3   Voluntary Euthanasia Society posters

out advertisements in journals and newspapers. The tactic does not seem to have been particularly successful. One hundred pounds was spent on advertising, and the posters brought in 'only' about 100 replies, a mere thirteen of which resulted in membership of the Society. The Society consoled itself with the comforting thought that the 'number of people who had discussed or considered the subject of euthanasia as a result were incalculable'.[33] This did not prevent the advertising campaign from being discontinued.

In the course of the year Dr MacDonald petitioned numerous MPs with a view to introducing a voluntary euthanasia Bill to the House of Commons, but without success. The most hopeful possibility had been Somerville Hastings, an MP who was also a doctor, but he felt unable to introduce the Bill on professional ethical grounds.[34] The former Honorary Secretary remarked in a letter to Miss Audrey Jupp that the problem of finding an MP to introduce the bill was not 'going to be at all easy'.[35]

A further and significant reason why the euthanasia movement failed to prosper during the 1950s was the emergence of the palliative care movement. In the early 1950s doctors could justifiably claim that literature on care of the dying was sparse.[36] Discussion of palliative care in cases of malignant disease centred around injections of morphine 'and some variation of the Brompton Mixture ... morphine, heroin and cocaine, given in whiskey or gin'.[37] Considerable progress was being made in palliative medicine.[38] By the late 1950s the work of individuals such as Cicely Saunders had gone some way towards undermining the case for voluntary euthanasia.[39] Saunders, a doctor, former nurse and medical social worker, advanced a 'remarkably far-sighted exposition of the varied elements of modern palliative care, discussing in turn the value of special homes for the dying and the need for attention to physical, spiritual, psychological and social problems'.[40] Improvements in the care of the dying purported to offer a direct alternative to euthanasia. If patients could die without acute pain and in a comforting environment there would be no need for euthanasia.

The impact of these changes on the case for euthanasia was recognised from within the Euthanasia Society. Certain individuals believed that the strength of the case for voluntary euthanasia was beginning to wane. Correspondence between Leonard Colebrook and the Chairman of the Society, Dr C. K. MacDonald, is particularly instructive on this point. Having being asked to take part in a debate on euthanasia, Colebrook became rather anxious when he began to think about how he would 'present or support the VELS thesis'.[41] Anticipating that his opponent would probably be a general practitioner, he recognised that one argument might be that because of developments in analgesia and a 'greater readiness to give plenty of dope in one form or another'[42] death need no longer entail protracted suffering. Colebrook's own experience with patients dying from tuberculosis, cancer, puerperal fever, and burns was mostly before 1940 and he was anxious not to present a picture which was 'out of date'.

> I see that in the Report of the VELS Mr Pollard says that 'the Society feels that the need for the bill becomes greater every year'. Is that really the situation if the means of relieving suffering are becoming more effective? ... I wonder whether we should not plead for the patient's right to relief when the need is less extreme, – for example in the many cancer cases in whom pain recurs every day for weeks or months and they only get relief from drugs when it becomes intolerable.[43]

Such concern seems to have prompted the Society to acquaint both itself and the public more explicitly with the dying experiences of the terminally ill.

The files of the Euthanasia Society abound with numerous case histories which seemed to show that unnecessary suffering was a logical concomitant of advances in life-prolonging medical technology. These case histories were explicitly sought by the executive committee because it was thought that they would serve as favourable propaganda.

In the course of 1959 Cicely Saunders had begun a series of six articles on the 'Care of the dying' which dealt with such subjects as: euthanasia; whether terminally-ill patients should be informed of their prognosis; nursing and control of pain in terminal cancer; and mental distress in the dying.[44] In one of these articles she had remarked that in 90 per cent of all cases she could keep suffering within bearable limits. This was a considerable achievement, but it also meant that in 10 per cent of cases 'approx. 9,000–10,000 cases a year with all her facilities' Saunders would be unable to render pain bearable. Colebrook believed that if the Society could 'produce a dozen or so of illustrative examples of terminal conditions in which euthanasia would have avoided great suffering' the Society's publication *Merciful Release* would be strengthened considerably.[45] Case histories were collected and subsequently featured in the Society's literature.

There is little doubt, however, that Saunders' articles served as powerful propaganda against the euthanasia movement. Her experience in two terminal homes indicated that the suffering of 90 per cent of the patients could be relieved. Patients were occasionally sedated, but importantly it was 'never' necessary to administer 'doses of narcotics which would be fatal in themselves'. She did not deny that some patients suffered, but claimed 'that the great majority need not do so'.[46] Although the administration of analgesics formed a central part of her approach, Saunders sought to pioneer an innovative and complete programme for the care of the dying which catered for the patient's mental and spiritual well-being as well as the amelioration of physical suffering. Thus, in addition to the application of local heat and antacids, 'attention to the bowels and all the other nursing treatments' could be useful in ameliorating severe pain.[47] Her approach was also underpinned by strong Christian faith. But for those whose sole concern was to minimise suffering, the suggestion that the last stages of a terminal illness offered the opportunity to become 'reconciled to God'[48] was a tangential and inadequate argument against euthanasia. Indeed, Saunders acknowledged that such 'transcendental reasons' carried little weight with the supporters of euthanasia. Nevertheless, she suggested further that the mechanisms for pain relief ensured that euthanasia could and 'should be unnecessary'.[49]

From the perspective of the euthanasiasts, however, the treatments administered to the dying under Saunders' supervision were the very sort which could be construed as denying the patient his dignity. Saunders' articles abounded with the sort of treatments which for the euthanasiast tormented the patient in his final moments, whereas a quick and merciful *coup de grace* could and should have been substituted. While some patients responded very favourably to 'reassurance, a careful diet and antacids'[50] there were others who were completely unable to tolerate any food, and instead survived on iced water or soda water. Others were forced to rely on sedatives and opiates in order to suppress vomiting fits induced by 'pain and misery'. Occasionally it was thought beneficial to insert a 'nasal tube' combined with 'intermittent or continuous suction to prevent the constant retching' and supplement the 'fluid intake with a rectal infusion'.[51] It was precisely the possibility of passing one's last days with a tube in every orifice that the euthanasiasts wished to avoid. Perhaps the majority of problems which afflicted the dying were amenable to treatment, but in many cases the treatments were detestable.

In particular cases of terminal cancer, dysphagia could be so severe that anything consumed by the patient would cause vomiting with a spill-over into the lungs. The administration of a local anaesthetic in gel form might ease this problem. Fungating growths were receptive to treatment with liquid paraffin. The patient's mouth might also be afflicted by the 'primary growth' in which case much pain could be avoided if kept scrupulously clean 'with frequent rinsing or syringing and any sepsis is treated with antiseptic paints or lozenges such as Dequadin or Hibitane. Local anaesthetic sprays or emulsions may be given before meals, but a patient may need a permanent nasal tube.'[52] 'The headache and vomiting of raised intracranial pressure may sometimes be relieved by magnesium sulphate enemas, diuretics or saline purgative if the patient is not already dehydrated.'[53] Urinary complications also posed a problem. Retention might make it necessary to insert an indwelling catheter. 'Patients with fistulae remain heavy nursing problems. Some wards use rubber bedpans and can keep patients comfortable and their backs intact; others prefer some kind of napkin. Silicone or local anaesthetic ointment will help to preserve the skin from excoriation'.[54] In fact Saunders acknowledged that these patients often felt 'humiliated' and therefore needed a great deal of 'reassurance and sympathy, they often need to be told that we do not mind dealing with these things'.[55] Similarly, the bowels were considered to be 'an everlasting source of interest and worry to fairly fit patients and may make life intolerable to the very ill. Impacted faeces must be removed, olive oil and water enema or suppositories may be needed and are less exhausting than strong purgatives, but if patients can be persuaded to take regular paraffin or emulsion these may be avoided.'[56] Asphyxia and dyspnoea

> are very hard to relieve and it may be impossible where the cause is obstructive. These patients rarely get any comfort from oxygen and hate almost any form of mask. Open windows are better if possible. Ephedrine and aminophylline will help where there is an element of spasm and are worth trying even when it gives no physical signs. Small doses of atropine will reduce sputum and may give

great relief to patients with tracheotomies, but the dose needs careful regulation.[57]

Although Saunders had pioneered a fairly comprehensive approach which certainly tempered the case for euthanasia, the respective approaches while having considerable overlap did not meet on exactly the same ground. For those patients who abhorred the prospect of losing their dignity and enduring significant discomfort, if not pain, Saunders' approach was commendable but unsatisfactory.

In addition to the emergence of the palliative care movement, intellectual engagement with the subject of euthanasia also began to increase at this time. Of particular note was the publication in 1955 of Joseph Fletcher's *Morals and Medicine*.[58] Fletcher was at the time professor of pastoral theology and Christian ethics at the Episcopal Theological School, Cambridge, Massachusetts. This book was a landmark text which opened up the whole field of medical ethics to intellectual, professional and public scrutiny. Prior to its publication, the 'extant' literature on medical ethics had consisted largely of 'homilies' concerning the physician's bedside manner, with much attention directed to 'such calculated questions of propriety and prudence as shined shoes, pressed trousers, tobacco odors, whether to drink Madeira, and the avoidance of split infinitives!'[59]

Fletcher's book dealt with a number of different medical ethical issues including the right of a patient to be told the truth by his doctor, birth control, sterilisation, artificial insemination, and euthanasia. The chapter dealing with euthanasia was particularly sympathetic. Offering a survey of the history and ethics of suicide, Fletcher employed a great deal of ethical reasoning to meet Christian objections to euthanasia on their own terms. It was noted, for example, that the Church had tolerated suicide when its purpose had been martyrdom or the retention of virginity. The core of Fletcher's argument, however, centred around his claim that the concern of the moralist was not with 'life qua life and its sacrosanctity, but with consciousness', a condition which was necessary for the 'patient's cooperation in last rights'.[60]

In previous chapters we have noted how different authors have justified their advocacy of euthanasia, the 'good death', by referring to different conceptions of worthwhile life. Put simply, euthanasia has been considered justifiable when a life lacks certain qualities which would otherwise make it worthwhile. Fletcher espoused a view which asserted the primacy of personality. '[S]elf-possession and personal integrity' were identified as two qualities which were prerequisites for the living of a worthwhile life. Incurable pain was capable of destroying both of these qualities.[61] Asserting his 'personalistic view of man and morals' Fletcher claimed that the prolongation of life for its own sake when life was bereft of the 'personal qualities of freedom, knowledge, self-possession and control, and responsibility' was in essence an 'attack' upon the 'moral status of a person'.

Fletcher also detected a contradiction at the heart of the Hippocratic Oath. The physician's obligation to prolong life and relieve suffering were not always compatible. Arguably, in certain cases narcotic pain relief was effecting euthanasia albeit without admission and few seemed to object to this practice. Espousal of the doctrine of double effect had become increasingly widespread in the euthanasia discourse of the twentieth century. Indeed, it had become such common currency that by 1957 even the resolute Catholic stance on the ethics of medical practice in cases of terminal illness had begun to soften. The first indication of this shift became apparent during a papal address to an audience of doctors on 24 February in Rome. In the course of this address Pope Pius XII outlined the stance of the Roman Catholic Church concerning the moral problems of pain and anaesthesia in response to questions submitted by the Italian Society of the Science of Anaesthetics.[62] The Pope was asked whether in cases of terminal illness it was lawful for the terminally ill to make use of analgesic drugs even if the amelioration of pain was accompanied by a 'shortening of life'. He had replied that 'if the dying man has fulfilled all his duties and received the last Sacrament; if medical reasons clearly suggest the use of anaesthetics; if in determining the dose the permitted amount is not exceeded; if the intensity and duration of this treatment is carefully reckoned and patient consents to it, then there is no objection: the use of anaesthetics is morally permissible'.[63] In a second address delivered on 9 September 1958 to the members of the Collegium Internationale Neuro-Psycho-Pharmacologicum, the Pope elaborated further on this issue. Explaining that euthanasia, meaning the deliberate provocation of death was 'condemned by morality' he conceded that 'if the dying patient agrees, it is lawful to use, with moderation, narcotic drugs which will allay suffering, but also bring about an earlier death'. Such a course of action was deemed excusable because the patient's death was not explicitly intended, but 'inevitable and appropriate reasons make measures which will hasten its coming acceptable'.[64] The doctrine of double effect was, however, not without its critics.

Alongside Fletcher's *Morals and Medicine*, the most important intellectual contribution to the euthanasia debate during this period came from the Quain Professor of Jurisprudence at the University of London, and a Vice-President of the Euthanasia Society, Glanville Williams. Williams was probably the twentieth century's most distinguished criminal lawyer. His arguments were deeply rooted in his philosophical utilitarianism and he was a champion of numerous liberal causes. He supported the rights of prisoners to starve themselves to death, homosexual law reform, and in his capacity as president of the Law Reform Association wanted abortion legalised.[65] Williams's views on euthanasia were first advanced at length in a paper entitled 'Voluntary euthanasia – the next step' delivered at the Annual General Meeting of the Euthanasia Society in 1955.[66] The theme of this speech was subsequently developed in a comprehensive text published in 1958 entitled *The Sanctity of Life and the Criminal Law*,[67] which in addition to its consideration of the question of euthanasia also addressed the issues of contraception, abortion and sterilisation; all of which Williams supported.

In terms of the ethical issues involved, there were numerous similarities between the work of Williams and Fletcher. With regard to the doctrine of double effect, however, they differed markedly. In Williams's view the doctrine served as a mechanism for practising euthanasia without admission. One could not claim with any justification that a physician who administered a narcotic overdose to a patient with the intention of ending life was 'guilty of sin', while a physician who administered the same drug in the same circumstances with the aim of relieving pain was not guilty provided that he kept his mind 'steadily off the consequences which his professional training teaches him is inevitable, namely the death of his patient'.[68] For Williams such a distinction was simply 'too artificial'. He noted that the same principle was used to 'salve the Catholic conscience in some cases of therapeutic abortion'. In cases of problematic childbirth it was excusable to kill the baby in order to save the mother's life. The death of the child would be considered an unfortunate and unintended consequence of preserving the mother's well-being.

Aware that his conduct will have two consequences, one good and one 'evil', the physician as a moral agent is 'compelled' to choose between acting and not acting by making an assessment of whether the 'good is more to be desired than the evil is to be avoided'. If this was what was meant by the principle of double effect, then Williams was prepared to endorse it. But if – and this was a rhetorical 'if' – it meant that the dilemma of making this moral choice could be avoided simply by keeping one's mind off the consequences, it could only 'encourage a hypocritical attitude towards moral problems'. Indeed in a legal context there was no difference between 'desiring or intending' a consequence arising from one's action, and continuing in that act with the full knowledge that the consequence will arise though not specifically desired. According to Williams it was more sensible to make use of the common law notion of 'necessity'. Faced with 'a choice between competing values' the ordinary rule is departed from in order to 'avert some great evil'. The physician would be justified in administering any quantity of narcotic substance necessary to alleviate pain, even though he knew that such an act would speed or indeed precipitate the patient's death. The legal 'excuse' was not the Catholic doctrine of double effect, but the legal doctrine of necessity, for the patient's pain could not be relieved without killing the patient.[69] As a professor of jurisprudence Williams's analysis was imbued with a strong legalistic dimension. As the law stood, euthanasia was considered to be suicide on the part of the patient and either murder or manslaughter on the part of the doctor. There was no instance, however, of a doctor being prosecuted for euthanasia in Great Britain. The legal position was assumed but had never been put to the test, and Williams thought most judges would deem this form of euthanasia permissible under the 'existing law'.

This analysis from one of the foremost legal scholars of his time was significant because it attempted to put to one side the doctrine of double effect. Williams considered that the oft-cited case of euthanasia where a patient's life would be cut short by a few hours or days by the administration of pain killing narcotics was not really that contentious. In such cases there were no prosecutions, and the practice was probably legal. The implication was that the doctrine of double effect had been used as a tactical debating point by some advocates of euthanasia; it was something of a smoke-screen. For

Williams the real issue concerned the situation where a physician anticipated 'matters by administering a fatal dose – say doubling the previous dose of morphine – in order to save the patient from dragging out a numbed, miserable and hopeless existence'. Under the existing law such a practice was prohibited. It was in this 'field' that a change in the law was to be considered. Although the case for saving patients from great pain received considerable support, there was significantly more disagreement about whether a patient whose pain could be ameliorated would be 'required to continue an artificial, twilight existence, in a state of terrible weakness, and subject perhaps to nausea, giddiness, extreme restlessness, misery or other afflictions which may not be regarded as strictly pain'. Williams's view was perfectly frank, he was proposing to kill patients who were enduring a miserable life, but whose death was by no means imminent.

Under this proposal no physician who had intentionally accelerated the death of a seriously ill patient would be liable to prosecution for 'murder, manslaughter or lesser offence against the person' unless it could be proven that the act was not committed in good faith with the patient's consent and with the intention of avoiding severe pain accompanying 'an illness believed to be of an incurable and fatal character'. If charged, the physician would be obliged to demonstrate that the patient was 'seriously ill', but the burden of proving bad faith would rest upon the Crown.

Embracing a hedonistic conception of worthwhile life, Williams suggested that euthanasia was a justifiable measure whenever the prospect of happiness in a particular life had evaporated. According to this reasoning, the terminally ill were not the only potential recipients; 'severely handicapped infants' might also be 'rightfully' put to death. Such a policy was some considerable way from securing the approval of popular opinion. As Williams lamented, there remained a tendency to 'regard all human life as sacred however disabled or worthless or even repellent the individual may be'.[70] A system of euthanasia for 'severely handicapped babies' would require the co-operation of the medical profession, which could not be guaranteed. The most practical option, therefore, was for the courts to regard 'the condition of the child killed' as the 'strongest mitigation of legal guilt'. Indeed, it was noted that the courts had already obtained considerable discretion to 'discharge without punishment' where this appeared to be 'expedient'. While not explicitly approving euthanasia of defective infants, Williams noted that toleration should be regarded as a virtue; he suggested that the mother's 'eugenic killing' of her child paralleled the 'bitch that kills her misshapen puppies'. The act could not 'confidently be pronounced immoral' and in the absence of such certainty, liberty should prevail.[71] In those instances where natural selection failed to operate quickly enough, Williams noted favourably that in Britain, doctors and nurses did not 'strive officiously to keep alive' seriously defective infants although they did not take any positive action to kill it. Left unattended for some time the malformed infant would usually die, unlike the normal infant who would usually survive.

The number of 'degenerate children' was said to be increasing and in the future mankind might be forced to adopt a 'policy of "weeding out" which is at variance with our present humanitarian outlook'.[72] Williams suggested that the Euthanasia Society had never advocated euthanasia for 'hopelessly defective infants'[73] and from an official perspective this was indeed true. But as we have seen throughout this book, such proposals had been voiced by numerous prominent figures within the Society. By the turn of the decade discussion of euthanasia for defective infants had become an even more prominent theme of the euthanasia debate. Sir Ronald Fisher, for example, President of Gonville and Caius College, Cambridge, was reported in *The Times* as having proposed euthanasia for 'seriously deformed or mentally deficient children'.[74] His proposal elicited numerous complaints from readers.[75]

A satirical letter to *The Lancet* in October of 1954 provides a particularly vivid example of the perceived problem resulting from medical advances which appeared to be extending the length of human life without due regard for its quality.[76] Babies whose birth weight was as small as three pounds could survive if they received intensive treatment in specialised units for the care of premature babies, combined with 'hours of devoted nursing', blood transfusions, antibiotics. Even so, the result could be a 'spastic diplegic idiot'. Intensive care for premature babies, particularly those with low birth weights ensured that there would be some who were 'better dead'. The letter noted that twenty years previously a baby with a birth weight of four pounds or less usually did not survive. Technological advance had modified this situation, but the author felt that this produced too many physically and mentally defective infants.[77] This letter sharply criticised the way in which the limited funds of the National Health Service were being allocated. In addition to criticising the lavish resources spent on neonatal care, the letter attacked the resources spent on geriatric care. To devote a high proportion of limited resources 'to rearing new citizens who will never support themselves, and on prolonging the lives of others who can only hope to leave their beds for their graves'[78] was of questionable logic. Thus the economic arguments which we have seen pervading the euthanasia debate from the late nineteenth century onwards, became still more relevant with advances in medical technology in the second half of the twentieth century. In a world of limited budgets the questions of economics and the ethics of medical treatment became more pressing, afflicting the National Health Service from its very inception.

> The hemiplegic of 85 with pneumonia – do you give antibiotics? The 90-year-old with a fractured neck or femur – do you pin? The mentally defective with nutritional anaemia – do you transfuse? The mongol with a congenital heart – do you operate? ... If we pursue our present course we must spend more and more on the care of mental defectives, on the training of spastics, and on geriatric beds, while the services for the working population are pressed ever tighter. ... if our present trends in birth and death-rates continue, an ever-decreasing proportion of workers must support an ever-increasing proportion of physically and mentally infirm. ... The trouble is that most of us feel more guilty about the unpleasant results of our actions than about the equally unpleasant results of our inactions.[79]

The development of medical technology had begun to complicate considerably the ethical issues surrounding euthanasia, and in so doing brought the whole question to the fore. Indeed it prompted a fundamental re-conceptualisation of death and notions of worthwhile life. As Fletcher remarked, '[t]he dimensions of our moral responsibility expand of necessity, with the advances made in medical science and medical technology. Almost every year brings with it some new gain in our struggle to establish control over health, life and death.'[80] Among these technological advances was the development of the respirator, an instrument which facilitated the artificial ventilation of patients whose respiratory system was unable to function independently. Other notable developments in the course of the 1950s included the use of generalised hypothermia which made possible intracardiac surgery along with the development of the heart–lung machine which facilitated artificial oxygenation of the blood.[81] Because of breakthroughs of this nature, the ethics of medical care needed to evolve and to 'engage constantly in self-correction'.[82]

The development of respirators and other life-prolonging techniques also complicated the definition of death.[83] The increasingly sophisticated nature of medical technology enabled physicians to drag out lives beyond the point at which until comparatively recently the individual concerned would have died promptly. As early as 1954 an article published in the *Medical Press* had suggested that the question of euthanasia or mercy-killing was becoming more pertinent because of these developments.[84] It noted that pneumonia had once been described not only as 'captain of the men of death', but as 'the old man's friend'. Pneumonia had carried off the aged with comparative speed, relieving them of a prolonged infirmity; providing 'euthanasia without presenting any moral or ethical problem to the doctor, cutting short many lives which were useless or burdensome'.[85] The development of antibiotics had complicated the issue considerably. Physicians felt they had to prescribe them, yet they knew that by doing so they would leave the patient to die more slowly from other afflictions. In fact the article noted that there was 'little hesitation about forgiving the doctor who does withhold them when pneumonia comes to a patient who is dying painfully by inches'.[86] Euthanasia was cautiously endorsed.

Speaking in 1954 about the 'problems of old people' the General Secretary of the Surrey Council of Social Service noted that because of the increasing number of the elderly, it was inevitable that the pensionable age would be raised in the future. He also remarked that 'medical science' had 'upset the balance of nature and the old law of the survival of the fittest ... In Iron Curtain countries euthanasia was being discussed because they consider the problem in completely ruthless terms.'[87]

Perhaps the most extraordinary example of this kind, however, came from within the upper echelons of the Euthanasia Society itself. The occasion was an address by Dr Leonard Colebrook 'On easeful dying, and the population problem' at the Annual General Meeting of 1959. Colebrook, a retired physician who had specialised in treating infection and burns,[88] noted that in the previous one hundred years the age distribution of Great Britain had been subject to profound change. During the 1870s 1 in 21 people were over the age of 65, a proportion which had remained largely unchanged by the beginning of the twentieth century. By 1921, however, the proportion over the age of 65 had risen to 1 in 16 and by 1950 to 1 in 10. By 1957 the figure was 1 in 8, and according to Colebrook if the prevailing trends were to continue no fewer than 1 in 6 of the population would be over 65 by 1977. Between 1900 and 1957 there had been a 38 per cent increase in the total population of Great Britain, while the proportion over 65 had increased by 250 per cent. The number of people over 65 had risen from 1.5 million to 5.25 million. This trend was placing an ever heavier burden upon the state as a consequence of medical and nursing services and pensions.

Yet, 'it was wrong to think that people who had survived to 65 had an increased expectation of life of any importance'.[89] Colebrook believed that the problem of old age threatened the national economy. It was to be hoped that, 'as time progressed and the reality of the situation started to be accepted, a robust realism would grow up among the elderly and they would realise that the mere length of life was not in itself desirable. It was quality of life, not its length which mattered.' In the future, individuals who had enjoyed a long and useful life would, he hoped, wish to die with dignity. Faced with failing eyesight and hearing, unable to watch television, listen to the radio, or talk 'reasonably to friends', individuals would begin to welcome the prospect of death. Crippled with arthritis and bronchitis, unable to do any more 'useful work', with the prospect of further deterioration and senility, elderly people would become steadily more dependent on friends and relatives. For these individuals it was suggested that a death with dignity would be infinitely preferable to eking out a useless existence in their twilight years. Developments in medical knowledge and the advent of antibiotics had produced a 'lamentable tendency' among a large number of the medical profession who were keeping 'people alive even if that "life" consisted of years of being bedridden or badly paralysed with failing faculties'. Colebrook hoped that in the future the medical profession might realise that the interests of these patients would be best served by enabling them to slip out of their torturous existence rather than striving 'officiously' to keep them alive.[90]

Dr Eliot Slater, another member of the Euthanasia Society and the foremost psychiatric geneticist of his time, raised similar concerns. Lecturing to the Euthanasia Society on 13 March 1958 on

'The biologist and the fear of death',[91] Slater drew attention to the way in which advances in medical technology were being wantonly employed without due regard for the best interests of the patient. He cited the example of a 76-year-old lady in a poor state of health who was suddenly taken ill with a stroke. The stroke left her paralysed down her right side and unable to speak. An ambulance was called, but 'by the time she was wheeled into the casualty ward she had breathed her last breath'. Intent on saving the patient, all the resuscitation equipment at the hospital's disposal was employed. For eighteen hours the patient's heart was kept beating and respirators kept her breathing artificially, though 'mercifully' the 'determined battle was fought in vain'. When the casualty officer had been asked why this was being done, he replied that he was not professionally obliged to ask such questions: his sole duty was to deploy all available resources to 'ward off death'. He remarked frankly that even if it had been feasible to save the patient's life 'only the shell of a human being, speechless, paralysed, and demented, would have remained'.[92]

Like Fletcher, Slater stressed the importance of quality of life as opposed to the 'mere prolongation of the automatic action of heart, lungs, and bowels. A few more hours of mental lucidity and capacity to communicate were in a different dimension from months of coma, dementia, or idiocy.' Death tended to be regarded in an almost neurotic way, it seemed to be the last taboo. '[J]ust as people's minds were in a bad way on the subject of sex at the beginning of this century until Freud had let some light into a dark cupboard, so now we had the same attitude towards death'.[93] But in Slater's opinion death was often 'a boon to the individual and a benefit to the race, by eliminating the worn out and those whose part had already been played'. Unless the sick and aged died soon after they had ceased to be self-supporting, 'the burden on society would become disastrous'.[94] These concerns stemming from demography and technology failed to rouse popular sentiment, but in the course of the 1960s they would return with a vengeance.

The early 1950s had witnessed a sharp decline in the fortunes of the British euthanasia movement. Progress had been stifled by a conservative moral climate, lack of interest from the medical profession and the general public, and an inadequate leadership which engendered a sense of drift. The death of Charles Killick Millard and

the diaspora of the original executive committee had been particularly important in this regard. While the relocation of the Society to
London headquarters offered new hope to the struggling movement it also proved rather disruptive. Matters were not helped by
the resignation of the new Honorary Secretary, R. W. Pollard, and
the consequent loss of direction. Further and significant difficulties
were presented by a number of factors outside the confines of the
Society. Perhaps most notable among these was the burgeoning
palliative care movement which seemed to offer a direct alternative
to voluntary euthanasia. The Society also found publicity hard to
come by. For much of the 1950s public interest in the cause was
negligible. However, the intellectual engagement of philosophers
and lawyers had begun to reveal the increasing ethical complexity
brought about by advances in medical science and this revealed
signs of a more promising future for the euthanasia movement. It
became clear that due to the development of life-prolonging technology and demographic patterns, more attention would be
directed to the care of the dying and euthanasia would feature
prominently in the forthcoming debate.

Notes

1   *BMJ*, 23 Dec. 1950, p. 1447.
2   *The Times*, 19 Oct. 1950, p. 4; BMJ, 9 Dec. 1950, p. 1319.
3   Barbara Brookes, *Abortion in Britain 1900–1967* (London, 1988) p. 134.
4   Ross McKibbin, *Classes and Cultures: England 1918–1951* (Oxford, 1998)
    pp. 321–7; Hugh David, *On Queer Street: A Social History of British
    Homosexuality 1895–1995* (London, 1997) pp. 153–8.
5   Arthur Marwick, *British Society Since 1945* (London, 1982).
6   Trevor Fisher, 'Permissiveness and the politics of morality', *Contemporary
    Record*, Vol. 7, No. 1, Summer 1993, pp. 149–65.
7   Brookes, *Abortion in Britain*, p. 151.
8   *Ibid.*, p. 147.
9   Fisher, 'Permissiveness', p. 151; David, *On Queer Street*, p. 188.
10 David, *On Queer Street*, p. 189.
11 Fisher, 'Permissiveness', p. 151.
12 McKibbin, *Classes and Cultures*, pp. 303–4.
13 CMAC/SA/VES/B.9 *Evening Chronicle*, 16 July 1954; *Catholic Times*, 9 July
    1954; *The Universe*, 9 July 1954.
14 CMAC/SA/VES/B.9 *Daily Dispatch*, 11 Dec. 1953.
15 CMAC/SA/VES/A.11 AR 1951.
16 Obituary, *Eugenics Review*, 1953, pp. 12–13.
17 CMAC/SA/VES/A.11 AR 1953.
18 CMAC/SA/VES/A.11 AR 1954.

19   *Ibid.*
20   *Ibid.*
21   CMAC/SA/VES/A.11 AR 1955, p. 7.
22   CMAC/SA/VES/A.11 AR 1954.
23   CMAC/SA/VES/A.11 AR 1954, p. 10.
24   *Ibid.*
25   *Ibid.*
26   CMAC/SA/VES/A.11 AR 1954, p. 7.
27   *Ibid.*
28   CMAC/SA/VES/A.11 AR 1955, p. 4.
29   *The Times*, 16 Feb. 1955, p. 5.
30   *Ibid.*
31   *The Times*, 13 Jun. 1955.
32   CMAC/SA/VES/o/s2/B.20.
33   CMAC/SA/VES/A.14 Minutes of the Twenty-second Annual General Meeting of the Euthanasia Society held on Thursday, 2 Apr. 1959.
34   CMAC/SA/VES/A.12 Letter from Somerville Hastings to Miss A. Jupp, 4 Oct. 1957.
35   CMAC/SA/VES/A.12 Letter from Robert Pollard to Miss A. Jupp, no date but surrounding documents indicate that the letter was written in Jun. 1957.
36   See for example: Clarence John Gavey, *The Management of the 'Hopeless' Case* (London, 1952).
37   *The Practitioner*, Vol. 177, 1956, p. 85.
38   See for example: S. Gerson, D. W. Bruce, N. Orchard, and F. H. Shaw, 'Amiphenazole and morphine in production of analgesia', *British Medical Journal*, 9 Aug. 1958, pp. 366–8.
39   Shirley Du Boulay, *Cicely Saunders: Founder of the Modern Hospice Movement* (London, 1984).
40   David Clarke, 'Someone to watch over me', *Nursing Times*, Vol. 93, No. 34, 20 Aug. 1997, p. 50.
41   CMAC/SA/VES/A.14 Letter from Leonard Colebrook, 18 Nov. 1957.
42   *Ibid.*
43   *Ibid.*
44   See *Nursing Times*, 9 Oct. 1959, pp. 960–1; 16 Oct. 1959, pp. 994–5; 23 Oct. 1959, pp. 1031–2; 30 Oct. 1959, pp. 1067–9; 6 Nov. 1959, pp. 1091–2.
45   CMAC/SA/VES/A.14 Letter from Leonard Colebrook to Dr C. K. McDonald, 30 Oct. 1959.
46   *Nursing Times*, 9 Oct. 1959, p. 961.
47   *Nursing Times*, 23 Oct. 1959, p. 1031.
48   *Nursing Times*, 9 Oct. 1959, p. 961.
49   *Ibid.*
50   *Nursing Times*, 6 Nov. 1959, p. 1091.
51   *Ibid.*
52   *Ibid.*
53   *Ibid.*
54   *Ibid.*, p. 1092.
55   *Ibid.*
56   *Ibid.*
57   *Ibid.*

58 Joseph Fletcher, *Morals and Medicine* (Princeton, 1955).
59 *Ibid.*, p. 6.
60 *Ibid.*, p. 182.
61 *Ibid.*, pp. 186–7.
62 See *The Times*, 25 Feb. 1957, p. 6.
63 *Ibid.*
64 Cited in I. Van Der Sluis, 'The movement for euthanasia 1875–1975', *Janus,* Vol. 66, pp. 131–72.
65 Williams's obituary, *The Daily Telegraph*, 16 Apr. 1997, p. 27.
66 CMAC/SA/VES/B.1.
67 Glanville Williams, *The Sanctity of Human Life and the Criminal Law* (London, 1958).
68 *Ibid.*, p. 286.
69 *Ibid.* pp. 287–91.
70 *Ibid.*, pp. 30–1.
71 *Ibid.*, p. 31.
72 *Ibid.*, p. 35.
73 *Ibid.*, p. 311.
74 *The Times*, 10 Apr. 1959, p. 12.
75 *The Times*, 13 Apr. 1959, p. 11; *The Times*, 17 Apr. 1959.
76 CMAC/SA/VES/B.9 'The Widdicombe File XVIII Quo Vadis?', *The Lancet*, 23 Oct. 1954.
77 *Ibid.*
78 *Ibid.*
79 *Ibid.*
80 Fletcher, *Morals and Medicine*, p. 11.
81 Louis J. Acierno, *The History of Cardiology* (New York, 1994) pp. 630–48.
82 Fletcher, *Morals and Medicine*, p. 26.
83 Peter Singer, *Rethinking Life and Death* (Oxford, 1995) pp. 20–37; J. L. Bernat, C. M. Culver and B. Gert, 'On the definition and criterion of death', *Annals of Internal Medicine*, 1981, Vol. 94, pp. 389–94.
84 *The Medical Press*, 18 Aug. 1954, pp. 147–8.
85 *Ibid.*, p. 147.
86 *Ibid.*
87 CMAC/SA/VES/B.9 *Epsom Herald*, 30 Apr. 1954.
88 *Who Was Who* CD ROM (1996).
89 CMAC/SA/VES/A.14 Minutes of the 22nd AGM of the Euthanasia Society, 'On easeful dying and the population problem' an address by Dr Leonard Colebrook, 2 Apr. 1959.
90 CMAC/SA/VES/A.14 AGM Minutes, 2 Apr. 1959.
91 *BMJ*, 12 Apr. 1958, p. 885.
92 *Ibid.*
93 *Ibid.*
94 *Ibid.*, p. 886.

7

The 1960s: quality versus quantity

During the 1960s the fortunes of the euthanasia movement were reversed. By the end of the decade a second Voluntary Euthanasia Bill had been introduced to the House of Lords. Ultimately the Bill was rejected, but it enjoyed a far more favourable hearing than the previous parliamentary excursions. This chapter seeks to explain the recovery of the euthanasia movement during this period. In so doing it suggests that the moral climate of the 1960s was far more propitious than that of the 1950s. The term the 'permissive society' is both well-established and instructive. This was an era of sexual liberation with widespread use of contraceptives, legalisation of homosexuality and a relaxation of censorship laws.[1] Important changes were also particularly marked with regard to questions of life and death. A succession of Acts implemented several of these changes.

In 1961 suicide was legalised, in 1965 the death penalty was suspended for a trial period of five years[2] before being abolished in 1969,[3] and in 1967 David Steel's Abortion Law Reform Bill provided legislative sanction for abortion on therapeutic grounds.[4] These reforms all seemed to enhance the freedom of the individual and consequently appeared to offer a window of opportunity to the euthanasia movement. The recovery of the movement was also aided by a set of more specific factors including a consistent leadership, shortcomings in palliative care, and most importantly advances in medical technology. Life-prolonging apparatus and techniques complicated considerably the ethical conundrums which had persistently accompanied discussions of euthanasia but which in the course of the 1960s became questions with enormous practical bearing. Concerns about the counter-selectivity of modern medicine were reinvigorated, and as a result discussion about quality of life as a consideration in questions of medical ethics was heightened.

This chapter concludes by offering a tentative account of why the attempt to secure legislative endorsement of voluntary euthanasia failed. In addition to the objections which had persistently dogged legislative reform in this area it is suggested that the increasing ethical complexity of the euthanasia debate made it possible to use rhetorical devices which either camouflaged or side-stepped the question of euthanasia and thereby negated the necessity for legislative reform.

During the 1950s the Euthanasia Society had been blighted with problems of leadership. In the following decade such difficulties were almost entirely absent. Although there were changes in personnel there was a large reservoir of experience upon which to draw. This ensured that no position was left vacant and there was no need to advertise for enthusiastic and suitable successors. In 1960 when C. K. MacDonald the chairman of the Society died he was replaced immediately by the long-serving Leonard Colebrook. Three years later when Colebrook himself suffered a heart attack Maurice Millard was able to step into the breach on a temporary basis. Millard held the position for a year before resigning because it was difficult for him to publicise the Society in his own name while still in practice. He was also suffering from poor health and so could not devote sufficient 'time and attention' to the work of the Society.[5] He was succeeded by the Revd A. B. Downing, a Unitarian minister and editor of the *Inquirer,* who had served on the executive committee of the Euthanasia Society since 1962. In 1964 Mr C. R. Sweetingham was appointed secretary. This enduring partnership ran the Society for the next ten years. Other prominent figures such as Glanville Williams, the well-known professor of jurisprudence, and Eliot Slater, the eminent psychiatric geneticist, continued to be active in the Society.

In the course of the late 1950s palliative medicine and the broader question of care for the dying had begun to receive far more attention than at any previous time. To some extent developments in this field seemed to undermine the case for euthanasia. Individuals such as Cicely Saunders were able to show that in a high proportion of terminal illnesses death could be made reasonably comfortable. The Euthanasia Society's own document *The Case for Voluntary Euthanasia* (1961) noted that although people's experience of death varied widely, a small number were fortunate to be cared for during their final days in specialist hospitals dedicated to making patients 'fairly comfortable' when cure was impossible. In the 'sympathetic and sometimes surprisingly cheerful atmosphere' created by a predominantly religious and devoted nursing staff, terminally-ill patients were 'gentled' along so that they might face death 'with a quiet mind – unafraid'. It was thought that few of these patients would 'wish to avail themselves' of euthanasia even if it were legalised. Because there were so few of these hospitals, however, the need for euthanasia remained. Most patients spent their final days at home or in hospital wards. Those dying at home could expect a daily visit from the district nurse who would provide what help she could but this would need to be supplemented by the help of 'relatives or friends, usually well-intentioned but not always skilful'. In the wards of often understaffed general hospitals 'acute and curable diseases' tended to take priority and in these circumstances the relief of suffering was often far from satisfactory. There had 'undoubtedly been progress in the conquest of pain, but that conquest' was by no means 'complete'.

Although the emergence of the hospice movement offered an alternative to euthanasia it also helped to advertise the problems associated with terminal illness and the variety of mechanisms for coping with these difficulties. This was underlined during the early 1960s by a number of empirical studies which assessed the pain and distress of the dying. Systematic studies had earlier been conspicuous by their absence. Despite confirming that significant progress had been made in palliative care these studies also lent some credence to the claims of the euthanasiasts.

In 1961 *The Lancet* published a particularly illuminating study based on 220 patients who were inpatients of a geriatric unit at the time of their death.[6] This study conducted by A. N. Exton-Smith, physician at the Widdington Hospital, noted that by employing analgesic drugs and radiotherapy it was possible to control pain in a high proportion of patients suffering from malignant disease. Over half were 'pain free' and the presence of carcinoma in six patients became apparent only at necropsy. Despite this, there were striking exceptions. Four patients suffered acute dyspnoea, dysphagia, nausea and vomiting. Another patient suffering from colon cancer with secondary carcinoma in the bone was riddled with pain for a period of sixteen weeks.

Among the patients with cardiovascular disease pain was even more pronounced. One patient 'whose distress lasted several months' asked repeatedly 'to be done away with'. In seven other cases severe dyspnoea and a feeling of suffocation caused 'obvious distress'. Analgesic drugs were similarly ineffective with regard to disorders of the central nervous system. Eleven patients were confined to chairs from between one and four years. Another patient suffering from paraplegia was confined to a chair for eight years and subsequently to bed for six months. Although their degree of distress was difficult to determine, the lives of these patients were thought to be 'almost totally devoid of enjoyment'. Dependence on relatives and nursing staff combined with the humiliating condition of incontinence compounded their sense of 'helplessness'.[7] At the time of their terminal illness 41 per cent of the patients were mentally confused. Many died from exhaustion. Aware that they were dying, several patients lost the will to live and hastened death by rejecting food. Eleven patients persistently expressed their wish to die. One patient thought that the doctors were doing too much to treat her, another 'asked to be done away with', and 'some prayed for death'. The study revealed clearly that pain, discomfort and distress still accompanied the deaths of a significant number of patients. Indeed the advent of modern anti-biiotic drugs which relieved conditions such as bronchopneumonia effectively precluded the swift *coup de grace* which had previously relieved so many terminally-ill patients.

These findings were reinforced by J. M. Hinton of the Middlesex Hospital, whose study confirmed that doctors were still unable to 'control all physical discomfort in the dying'.[8] Mental distress was 'sufficiently common for a significant number of patients to consider suicide'.[9] Having assessed the physical and mental condition of 102 patients dying in hospital compared with patients suffering from serious but non-fatal illnesses, Hinton observed that the 'dying had a significantly higher incidence of unrelieved distress. They were more commonly depressed (45 per cent) and often anxious (37 per cent)'.[10]

In many cases physical pain could be relieved by drugs, but the accompanying problems of breathlessness, persistent vomiting, difficulty of swallowing, insomnia, bed-sores, incontinence, blindness and deafness could all 'contribute to a very unhappy end to life'. There was a clear and incontrovertible need for more specialist hospitals, but these institutions did not negate the case for euthanasia; they were not direct substitutes. So the Euthanasia Society remained committed to secure 'for the minority whom medical science' was unable to palliate, 'the right to choose a humane curtailment of their misery when that becomes too hard to bear'.[11] To this extent the euthanasia debate of the early 1960s did not significantly change. The inadequacy of therapeutic medicine in relieving the suffering of the dying remained the focus of discussion. From this point on, however, subtle shifts began to emerge in the debate which seem to have been responses to a series of contemporaneous events which all had some bearing on assessments of quality of life.

The legalisation of suicide in 1961 provided the first formal recognition of an individual's right to determine his own criterion of when life was no longer worthwhile. Indeed the Suicide Act seemed to foster the notion of a right to die.[12] One might have assumed, therefore, that legislative reform of euthanasia would have followed quickly. But the Act was a rather mixed blessing for the euthanasia movement. The Euthanasia Society tabled an amendment that would have exempted a compassionate doctor from punishment if he assisted a suicide with the intention of relieving suffering but it was not adopted. Consequently, Kenneth Robinson's Bill, though decriminalising suicide, carried a prison sentence of up to fourteen years for those convicted of assisting a suicide. The legal censure of euthanasia was thus reinforced. Furthermore, in removing from the criminal sphere those who wished to end their lives, the Suicide Act probably went some way to diminishing the need for euthanasia. But suicide was not a viable option for everyone. As the Society noted, for 'many courageous spirits', particularly those suffering from paralysis, release by suicide would not be possible without assistance from a physician. At this stage the Society's legislative proposals maintained that euthanasia would not be administered except in cases of illnesses which were 'likely to prove fatal in the not-distant future' and which were the cause of suffering that could not be relieved.[13] This stipulation was later dropped.

During 1962 interest in euthanasia returned in earnest. Once again a legal case provided the spark. On this occasion, however, it was neither the assisted suicide of a terminally-ill patient nor the parental killing of a mentally defective child. The case in Liége, Belgium concerned the murder charge and subsequent acquittal of the parents of a physically defective infant. Carine Vandeput's deformities were caused by thalidomide, a sedative which had been championed as a 'wonder sleeping pill' with no side effects. The drug had been recommended particularly for pregnant women suffering from morning sickness. This recommendation had been made without any knowledge of 'whether or not the drug crossed the placenta, thereby reaching the embryo inside the womb'.[14] The result was that worldwide somewhere in the region of 8,000–9,000 babies were born with pronounced physical deformities.[15] Approximately 500 thalidomide-impaired babies were born in Britain with a survival rate of around 50 per cent.[16] The case generated a huge amount of press coverage which seems to have served as a considerable fillip to the euthanasia movement.

The Times published no less than forty-five letters relating to the Vandeput case. A great deal of the press material was favourable to the parents. Readers' letters spoke of the 'agony' endured by parents caring for a 'crippled child'. This was considered to be a 'martyrdom to which no human being should be subjected'. The family had taken the law into their own hands because this was the only merciful course of action open to them. In order to prevent an increase in the 'vast sum of human misery' there was considerable support for the idea of killing 'grotesquely deformed' babies. 'Common sense, common experience and common humanity all counsel such a course; ranged against it is the grim trio of dogma, doctrine and taboo.'[17] Indeed proposals for 'legalized euthanasia' were explicitly advanced.[18] Repeatedly it was suggested that the right to life applied only to cases where life was 'normal' and 'healthy'. Life should not be maintained 'at any price'. This view seemed to have been endorsed by the Belgian jury 'who being human, were able to distinguish between "condemn to live" and "preserve the right to life"'.[19] This was not one of the more typical cases of euthanasia but it had raised the issues of quality of life and mercy-killing in a particularly vivid and public fashion. While the case was not strictly within its terms of reference, the Euthanasia Society felt that it had 'brought home to very many people all over the world the whole problem in a way that had not happened before'.[20]

Considering that the number of babies impaired by thalidomide was actually rather small when compared to the total of approximately 15,000 defective babies born annually in Great Britain[21] the effect of the tragedy was quite disproportionate. It had been far more successful in arousing interest and discussion than the more numerous cases of 'monstrous or defective infants'.[22] Nevertheless, the publicity which the case enjoyed gradually focused attention on to this larger group which in turn raised concerns about the counter-selectivity of medicine and the profile of quality of life judgements in questions of medical ethics.

The increasing preoccupation of the medical profession with these issues was indicated by the fact that the Royal Society of Medicine organised a symposium on 'The cost of life'[23] which discussed such issues as haemodialysis, organ transplantation, severe head injuries, tetraplegia, malformed infants, the mentally subnormal, the elderly and the sanctity of life. Medical ethics had been complicated considerably by recent developments in medical technology. In the course of his address on 'The community's responsibilities to the malformed child', Thomas McKeown, Professor of Social Medicine at the University of Birmingham, noted that between 1954 and 1963 the number of severely defective patients in sub-normality hospitals had increased by 6,500. Some of this increase could be attributed to greater institutional provision, but the advances in 'medical and surgical practice' which had improved survival rates were another important factor.[24] In particular cases, modern technology could prolong lives which previously would have ended in days or weeks. There was also a recognition that particular lives were bereft of value, though little consensus about the methods and legitimacy of effecting a premature death.

The medical profession as a whole had persistently opposed the deliberate killing of patients, but the idea that the doctor was not always obliged to prolong life was entertained more readily. Of course to abstain from a particular course of treatment and/or care would have the same result as a lethal injection – the individual would die, albeit more slowly – but for many, the concept of omission seemed to be morally less culpable than a direct action. The distinction between killing and allowing to die has not secured universal endorsement. Indeed, just as Glanville Williams had identified the doctrine of double effect as a rhetorical device for committing camouflaged euthanasia, there are grounds for thinking that the active–passive distinction has been used as another mechanism for avoiding a moral dilemma despite effecting death when it is thought desirable. These were subtle shifts in the euthanasia debate which were responses to the increasing complexity of medical treatment.

Surgical innovations had a particularly marked effect on mortality rates in cases of spina bifida and as a result discussion of appropriate treatment was especially contentious. In comparison to the number of defective births caused by Thalidomide, spina bifida was quite common, affecting approximately two live births per thousand.[25] In its more pronounced form, known as myelomeningocele, the baby's back has a swelling which leaks spinal fluid. The infant's spinal nerves are damaged and there is considerable risk of infection. For those who survive, paralysis in the legs is probable. Deformities of the spine are common and incontinence usual. In approximately 65 per cent of cases hydrocephalus develops. As a result a high proportion of children with spina bifida suffer brain damage.[26] Before the development of antibiotic drugs the prevalence of spinal infection ensured that few spina bifida babies survived. The combination of antibiotics, a surgical operation to close the spinal wound, the insertion of a tube under the skin of the head allowing cerebro-spinal fluid to be withdrawn and the advent of the Holter cranial valve in 1955, which alleviated the problem of persistent blockages, meant that for the first time life for spina bifida infants became a realistic possibility. By the early 1960s it had become possible to prolong the lives of babies afflicted with this condition, but there was considerable debate about the desirability of doing so. The three options which seem to have been contemplated were: (1) to kill the baby; (2) to withhold treatment and feeding; (3) to employ all means available to prolong the baby's life.[27] The most forceful advocate of the third option was R. B. Zachary, consultant paediatric surgeon at the Children's Hospital Sheffield. In his view all babies with severe myelomeningocele should be encouraged to live despite the fact that the majority would be 'severely handicapped'.[28] In fact surgery for spina bifida babies did become a matter of course during the 1960s.

This policy of active treatment, however, encountered strong criticism, and Eliot Slater would take a particularly active role in this debate during the early 1970s.[29] A decision to undertake surgery might ensure survival but there was no prospect of a normal life for the child. Ten per cent would be permanently confined to a wheelchair, others would need to use a chair for much of the time and the remainder would require callipers. Hydrocephalus could be controlled in many cases but revision operations might be necessary.[30] A child with spina bifida could expect to undergo up to forty orthopaedic operations in addition to the operations required to rectify problems with the drainage tube and urinary bypass operations. These procedures were particularly onerous for the patient. There was serious doubt about whether they produced an acceptable quality of life for the recipient and they were also expensive. In addition to medical expenses there were substantial educational costs.[31] The idea of non-intervention, letting 'nature take its course' attracted numerous supporters.[32] This was in effect a passive form of euthanasia, and for many among the medical profession this was ethically acceptable.

Defective babies and their improved rates of survival were not the only reason why these concerns had become more pertinent. The broader category of mental incapacity presented comparable dilemmas. Between 1948 and 1966 the mortality rate from acute head injury declined from 9 per cent to 3.5 per cent. The use of antibiotics, blood transfusions, 'the identification of metabolic disorders and their correction, and the newer therapeutic weapons such as hypothermia and cerebral hypotensive agents' had all combined to improve results. Although these methods of treatment ensured that a high proportion of patients could survive and make an 'excellent recovery', there were others 'for whom the price of life' was 'permanent invalidism'.[33] In these cases the desirability of further treatment was far from certain.[34] Quality of life seemed to be very poor and the medical and nursing demands combined with the cost of treatment were very heavy.[35]

In an article entitled 'The prolongation of dying' *The Lancet* drew attention to cases in which the human brain was effectively destroyed leaving the patient incapable of consciousness or communication, but able to survive as a functioning organism because particular activities could be 'mediated by the diencephalon and brainstem'.[36] In order to keep alive 'such fragmentary creatures' it would be necessary to employ a skilled medical team. In addition to placing heavy demands on nursing care, laboratory resources would also be required to conduct 'biochemical and bacteriological investigation'.[37] It was considered futile to prolong the husks of human life and this was underpinned by an economic rationale. The article noted that:

If the average length of a patient's stay in hospital is two weeks, a bed in that hospital occupied by an unconscious patient for a year could have been used by 26 other patients, whose admission has been correspondingly delayed. Apart from the addition to human suffering which this involves, the life of one or more of these 26 could actually have been lost through delay in obtaining necessary treatment. In a country without a surplus of hospital beds, an irrevocably unconscious patient may sometimes be kept alive at the cost of other people's lives.[38]

We have seen that among the medical profession the dilemma between preserving life or the quality of life was becoming increasingly acute. Such concern fed back into the Euthanasia Society which in turn began to reappraise the nature of its proposals. At the Society's Annual General Meeting of 1966 a memorandum was read which would have altered significantly the Society's policy had its proposals been adopted. It suggested that the Society's existing policy of a 'restricted form of euthanasia', was rather 'cumbersome', it had failed to 'rouse effective popular support' and it left entirely out of consideration 'the plight of innumerable sufferers who cannot make their wishes known or who are considered to be legally incapable of a reasoned appeal to mercy'. It was suggested that the Society should 'delete' from its proposals 'a word so manifestly inappropriate and so cruelly restrictive as "voluntary"'. Instead it should move resolutely 'towards a broad scheme of legislation based upon the whole range of the subject, abjuring the timidly clinical approach which, we may think, is hopelessly out of step with our times'.[39] This was the first indication of a shift in the Society's policy. Such a proposal had profound implications for defective babies, patients suffering from severe head injuries, and senile old people.

Indeed, the third and numerically most significant group for whom these issues were especially pertinent was the elderly. Numerous commentators alluded to the feelings of unease, 'if not revulsion, at the spectacle of some stuperous ancient in a hospital being maintained in a state of suspended animation by all the sophisticated paraphernalia of modern resuscitation'.[40] Although life-saving drugs and techniques were being employed quite properly for the young with 'intact brains', the ethics of administering the same treatments to the elderly were less clear. '[I]n many instances', such treatment was an 'ultimate disservice' to the old.[41]

Under the title 'Black cloud of senility' *The Observer* published a host of readers' letters which bemoaned the fact that increased longevity, aided and abetted by developments in medical technology, was often the cause of unacceptably low quality of life. Letters recorded the 'dread' with which the prospect of a 'useless, unhappy and unsavoury' life approached. There was hope that the time would come when public opinion was 'sufficiently enlightened to give elderly people the right and the means to opt out of life'.[42]

Economic considerations reinforced these arguments. The opportunity costs of treatment were rehearsed in some detail. It was noted that a disproportionate share of scarce National Health Service resources was being spent upon the elderly, which worsened the service for the young. In 1901 1.5 million people comprising 5 per cent of the population in England and Wales were over 65. In 1966 this had risen to 6 million, some 12 per cent of the population. The number over the age of 85 had increased from less than 50,000 to nearly 350,000 over the same period.[43] The per capita National Health Service expenditure on people over 65 was estimated to be approximately three times that expended on those below this age. The elderly were considered to 'consume more doctors' and nurses' time, more hospital beds, more operating theatre time, and above all more medicines than any younger group'. These facts had to be 'set against the recent cuts in, for example, school children's milk and the postponement of the raising of the school-leaving age'.[44] With a high proportion of the elderly afflicted by varying degrees of physical and mental ill-health a disproportionate burden was placed upon medical and social services. This provided a strong 'challenge to the public conscience'. Indeed, it raised the difficult question of what proportion of society's assets could and should be devoted to 'that percentage of the population which is steadily increasing, which cannot of itself contribute to the national budget, but is in turn entirely dependent on it'.[45]

The notion that human life was not always worth prolonging seems to have been gaining considerable ground. Public interest in this issue also seems to have proliferated at this time. Of particular note were a number of news reports concerning a notice posted in the Neasden Hospital in London instructing staff that 'in cases of cardiac arrest certain categories of patients were not to be resuscitated – those over 65; and those with malignant diseases or chronic chest or kidney diseases. These patients were to have their medical treatment cards labelled 'NTBR – Not To Be Resuscitated'.[46] This was certainly a controversial policy and the glare of publicity seems to have contributed to the removal of the notice after a period of sixteen months display. The Minister of Health was said to have been shocked and the *International Herald Tribune* carried the head-line 'Britain in Uproar over "Let Die" Directive'[47] but reactions were far from uniform.[48] *The Spectator* remarked that attempts to build the Neasden Hospital incident into a scandal had been 'unsuccessful' because there was 'a widespread feeling that there was sound common sense in a policy that allowed certain groups of patients to die in peace'.[49] A committee appointed to investigate the Neasden incident 'commended' the Physician Superintendent for attempting to deal with an 'appalling problem'. He was reprimanded, however, 'for being so indiscreet as to let the harsh truth disturb the compla-cency of a public which prefers to pretend such problems don't exist'.[50] In response to the incident the Euthanasia Society issued a press notice which suggested that in the case of a patient for whom resuscitation would bring little more than 'prolonged suffering' there should be a right to die. This policy received codification in the Society's draft bill of 1967 which formed the platform for the Bill of 1969. The Society noted that the 'wishes of the patient should always be of paramount consideration, and that once they have been clearly expressed they should be acted on, or at least respected, by all humane and conscientious persons having charge of the patient when he is in a helpless and pitiable condition'.[51]

Following the Neasden Hospital exposé the *Observer* published a two-part inquiry which drew attention to the sometimes officious approach of the medical profession. The first of these articles dealt with the pitiful case of a 70-year-old stroke victim. Conscious of the life which lay ahead he wrote 'laboriously' on a pad 'Let me die'. His wishes were ignored and he was kept alive unable to speak and paralysed down one side of his body. He suffered from inconti-nence, bed-sores, bladder problems, recurrent urinary infections and bouts of pneumonia. According to his doctor he was a 'human wreck'. He survived in this state until he was 85 when death finally 'released him'. As a result the man's doctor was converted to the case for euthanasia.[52]

Perhaps the most forceful example of this kind was a letter printed in the *British Medical Journal* which described in considerable detail the protracted death of a 68-year-old retired doctor in a foreign hospital.[53] The doctor was suffering from the advanced stages of cancer with 'extensive metastatic involvement of the abdominal lymph nodes and liver'. A palliative gastrectomy was performed in order to avoid perforating the primary tumour into the peritoneal cavity. Further investigation indicated that there were secondary deposits elsewhere in the body. The patient was informed of the pessimistic prognosis. Despite regular administration of large doses of pethidine and morphine he suffered persistent and acute abdominal pain and pain 'arising from the compression of spinal nerves caused by tumour deposits'.[54] After undergoing pulmonary embolectomy the patient requested that in the event of cardiovascular collapse no further efforts should be made to prolong his life because his pain was unbearable. Despite this he was resuscitated on no less than five occasions. He survived for a further three weeks 'in a decerebrate state, punctuated by episodes of projectile vomiting accompanied by generalized convulsions'. He was fed intravenously and received blood transfusions. Anti-bacterial and anti-fungal antibiotics were administered to prevent infection from complicating the tracheotomy which had been performed to secure clear airways. 'On the last day of the illness preparations were being made for the work of the failing respiratory centre to be given over to an artificial respirator, but the heart finally stopped before this endeavour could be realized.'[55] The publication of such disconcerting stories prompted intense discussion about the uses and abuses of modern medicine. Articles of this kind sought to stress that quality of life was far more important than its length. Scientific advance enabled the physician of a well-resourced hospital to maintain a condition that could be 'called "life" after most of the power, attributes and enjoyments of life have disappeared'.[56]

Before 1960 discussion about euthanasia had been concerned almost exclusively with those patients whose suffering medicine was unable to relieve. Thereafter, the discussion centred increasingly on cases where medical technology was able to prolong life but with poor quality. In this context medicine was perceived to be doing too much rather than too little. The 'knowledge, apparatus and skill' at the disposal of modern medicine had become 'so formidable' that serious questions were raised about the desirability of their use. As we have seen in the preceding discussion, the question of 'striving officiously to keep alive' had become a central feature of a more complex euthanasia debate. New and pressing questions of practical ethics included the point at which a patient should be allowed to die, and the point at which a patient could be pronounced 'dead'.[57]

Before the 1960s the biological concept of human death was fairly uncontentious. Thereafter the development and successful deployment of resuscitation techniques ensured that the cessation of breathing could no longer provide conclusive evidence of death. Similarly, the use of cardiac massage and the re-starting of the heart during cardiac surgery meant that curtailment of the heartbeat was no longer such a clear indicator of death. It was also well known that breathing could 'continue spontaneously for long after the central nervous system ha[d] decomposed or been destroyed beyond any known possibility of repair'.[58] The practical importance of these issues was illustrated by a number of articles published in the medical press which recorded the astonishing fashion in which lives seemingly lost were rescued by medical science.

The case of a five-year-old boy who was revived after drowning in a freezing river was cited as an example. Mouth-to-mouth resuscitation, external heart compression, a blood transfusion and injections restored the independent functioning of the boy's heart and lungs two hours after he had apparently died. On five occasions thereafter it was necessary to restore his breathing with artificial respiration and he needed to be fed intravenously for a week. After this he was able to swallow and rapidly regained his powers of recognition and comprehension. 'By all the standards of judgement employed up to the most recent times, this child would have been pronounced dead at a very early stage. Was he, in fact, "alive" or "dead" in those first two and a half hours?'[59]

The margins between life and death had narrowed considerably and advances in medical technology had made it necessary to reappraise the purposes of medicine in a fundamental way. In the course of his Harveian Oration to the Royal College of Physicians in 1965 Sir Theodore Fox had dealt explicitly with this issue.[60] He noted that whenever there was the possibility of genuine recovery the physician was right to preserve life by all the means at his disposal even though this might cause pain; his 'cruelty' was a 'kindness'. But to prolong a life which could 'never again have purpose or meaning' was senseless. The use of artificial respirators on a temporary basis with the clear intention of restoring a patient to independent breathing was uncontentious. They would be used merely to 'win time for restorative measures to take effect'. But if these techniques failed to produce the desired effect and it became apparent that the patient could never be restored to independent functioning, their continued use would keep the patient 'in a condition of artificially arrested death rather than "alive"'. In these circumstances the doctor might be justified in curtailing his use of the respirator in the same way that it had always been considered appropriate to curtail the older form of artificial respiration if this was proving ineffective.

Although many doctors and nurses felt that to abstain from efforts that might save a patient were tantamount to killing, the matter was one of degrees. Fox discussed the case of a patient dying 'miserably' from cancer who then acquired bronchopneumonia; although it would be wrong to precipitate the patient's death by withholding nourishment, it would be 'equally wrong', if the patient wanted to die, to prolong his suffering by prescribing antibiotics. There was a need to distinguish the 'desirable' from the 'feasible'. The physician was not the 'servant' of 'race', 'science' or even the servant of life, his obligations were to the 'individual interest' of his patient. 'With this mandate, he will remember that there is a time to live, but also, for all of us, a time to die. If possible with dignity.'[61]

It was in this context that the concept of 'ordinary' and 'extraordinary' methods of treatment was developed. 'Ordinary' treatment refers to that which a patient could 'obtain and undergo without thereby imposing an excessive burden on himself or others'. 'Extraordinary' treatment has been defined as 'whatever here and now is very costly or very unusual or very painful or very difficult or very dangerous or if the good effects that can be expected from its use are not proportionate to the difficulty and inconvenience that are entailed'. This distinction seems to have been formulated largely in response to the 'can-do, will-do technological imperative'.[62]

There was increasing consensus that the doctor was not always obliged to provide extraordinary treatment. But in cases where a patient, in a state of unconsciousness or 'vegetative existence' with no prospect of recovery, was kept alive simply by means of ordinary care rather than a plethora of technological devices the precise action which the doctor should take was rather unclear. Was the doctor obliged to feed the patient? There were grounds for thinking that if a doctor or nurse were to withhold food they would be guilty of negligence. If the patient subsequently died they would be liable for either manslaughter or murder. They would be similarly liable if they did not administer a readily available antibiotic. Again, if they turned off an artificial respirator deliberately they could be charged with murder, while to 'allow it to stop from neglect could well be manslaughter'.[63] But if one was able to argue that the best interests of a patient in a coma were not served 'while still debarred by Law from killing,' the doctor 'need no longer strive officiously to keep alive.'

In 1967 Chancellor E. Garth Moore, discussing the legal aspects of one's duty to the sick, noted that 'though the Law does not permit a direct act of killing, it may be that it does permit the withholding of the means necessary to keep the patient alive, and there would seem to be no valid distinction in principle between these different means, whether they be nourishment, antibiotics or the electric current which operates the apparatus for breathing'.[64] At this time there was no clear resolution of these issues, but their discussion highlighted medical ethics and euthanasia.

At the Euthanasia Society Annual General Meeting of 1968 a resolution was moved to the effect that pending the legalisation of voluntary euthanasia, patients found to be beyond 'remedial surgery' should be given strong sedatives but nothing else, intravenous feeding, in particular, was to be withheld. This controversial resolution was not adopted.[65]

Public exposure to the question of euthanasia also increased markedly at this time. On Saturday 27 May 1967 the BBC screened a programme in the 'Your Witness' series entitled 'Mercy Killing'. The programme took the form of a debate between Leo Abse MP and Professor Glanville Williams. Unfortunately from the perspective of the Euthanasia Society, the motion to be debated which was initially to have been 'euthanasia' was changed to 'mercy killing should no longer be a criminal offence'.[66] In the course of the programme Glanville Williams concerned himself with the question of ending the lives of the terminally ill. Leo Abse who opposed the motion concentrated his address 'almost exclusively' on the issue of 'deformed and defective children'. Consequently the two speakers never really met head on.

According to the Euthanasia Society this failure to concentrate on the issue of voluntary euthanasia ensured the defeat of the motion, which was lost by twenty-one votes to eight. Nevertheless the Society reported that the programme had been very 'worthwhile', as it had made 'millions' aware of the cause. It had brought about 'many enquiries, requests for speakers, and an encouraging number of new members. Above all, it has given great encouragement to us to continue our actions.'[67] The programme had received considerable and sympathetic coverage in the press. *The Observer* noted that Mr Leo Abse MP 'came across as a histrionic dandified farceur whose style of oratory, with its phoney legal phraseology, finger wagging, and deliberately playing for easy applause, showed up the hideous unreality of parliamentary emotionalism at its very worst'.[68] Euthanasia was also discussed on the David Frost Programme on ITV, 'when only 9 out of an audience of 150 opposed the action of a doctor who administered euthanasia at the request of an elderly, dying patient.'[69]

In the same year Dr Eliot Slater (Editor-in-Chief of the *British Journal of Psychiatry* and Director of the Psychiatric Genetics Unit of the Medical Research Council), a member of the Euthanasia Society executive committee, was interviewed by the BBC about euthanasia for a programme which was broadcast on the Overseas Service. Slater remarked that in the past ten years 'revolutionary technological advances' had been made 'which would enable spare parts or machinery to replace the functioning of organs that had ceased to work'.[70] He noted that dying and severely handicapped patients could be kept alive for weeks or even months with the aid of technology. This raised a concomitant ethical/moral question however. '[H]ow far it was right to keep people alive whose existence is very far from normal – whose brain, perhaps, had been so damaged as to reduce the victim almost to a vegetable state.'[71]

Occasionally there was a tendency to exaggerate what was medically possible, but the vista of surgical possibilities was indeed increasing rapidly. Of particular note in this regard was the first transplantation of a human heart performed by Dr Christian Barnard at the Groote Schuur Hospital in Cape Town on 3 December 1967. Such events indubitably had an important bearing on medical ethics and the question of how one should balance the desire to preserve life with the desire to secure an acceptable quality of life for one's patient. The apogee of this technology associated concern was an article entitled 'Transplantation and human rights' published in 1968. Making forays into science fiction the article noted that:

> Dr Barnard's world famous heart transplantation was the starting signal for an international race with no defined finishing line. After hearts, kidneys, lungs, liver, pancreas, what next? According to Dr Robert J. White, professor of neuro-surgery at the Cleveland General Hospital in America, it may be possible by the year 2001 to remove an undamaged brain from a body that has become useless through injury or disease and transfer it to a person who has died slowly of brain complications.
>
> ... The possibilities seem limitless. Could we be kept going, like an old car, by having a human replacement engine, gear-box or transmission fitted periodically? What effect would a new brain have on personality? Would the recipient take over the characteristics of the deceased donor? Would a living Mr Smith really be the late Mr Jones? Is the secret ambition no less than the conquest of death itself? The imagination boggles.
>
> Dr Murray Tondon of Stanford University has expressed what many must feel: 'The right to die may one day need to be defended as the most fundamental of human rights.' Some of us believe that that time has already arrived.[72]

In the course of a discussion about heart transplant operations with Dr Christian Barnard broadcast on the BBC's 'World at One' programme on 29 April 1968, Dr Donald Gould remarked that 'people have to die and under certain circumstances it is probably better to leave them to die in dignity, in peace, rather than to undertake heroic operations which have a small chance of success'. Asked whether it was not a doctor's job to try and save life wherever possible, Dr Gould said that this was becoming an increasingly difficult question to answer and on which to establish clear guidelines.

> We can now make it impossible for a person to die and the profession as a whole is beginning to realise that simply following this simple old rule that you just save life and put that as your principal aim isn't going to work any more because you can, you know, produce a living death: ultimately and ideally it should be the patient's choice but the patient has got to be able to appreciate what's going on. It is difficult to allow him to do that.[73]

Concern about the rights of patients had become so pronounced that organisations other than the Euthanasia Society began to adopt resolutions. In 1968 the British Humanist Association noting that advances in medical science enabled the aged and infirm to be kept alive for long periods ... sometimes against their will' passed a resolution calling for the 'early legislation of voluntary euthanasia'. In the same year the National Council for Civil Liberties and the National Secular Society both passed resolutions at their annual conferences which called attention 'to the natural right of individuals to seek euthanasia for themselves when their lives become intolerable, and for their doctors to be able to help them without risking a criminal prosecution'.[74]

Despite the broad shift in opinion towards euthanasia strong opposition persisted. For some the permissive environment of the 1960s seemed to be ushering in a concerted assault upon moral standards. This prompted some moral backlash. A letter from Miss E. Rhys Williams, Honorary Secretary of the Society for the Protection of the Unborn Child, provides a graphic example.

> May I inform your reader that, in view of a Bill having been prepared to legalise euthanasia, to be sponsored as were the Homosexual and Abortion Bills, by Humanists (atheists), a Society is being formed to oppose legalised euthanasia for the old or sick and sterilisation of the handicapped and unfit.
>
> Humanists, like Communists, do not believe in God or a Hereafter, they describe purity, innocence, and restraint as 'barren virtues.' ... Those who follow the 'permissive society' can find no real happiness in life. One has only to look into the tortured faces of young drug addicts. God help them: This 'permissive' government has a lot to answer for.[75]

Similar concerns were expressed in the Catholic press to the effect that the Abortion Act may have 'opened legal and medical doors to a new Bill promoting the legalisation of voluntary euthanasia'.[76]

In 1967 the Euthanasia Society published a new draft bill drawn up by Miss Mary Rose Barrington, a barrister and a member of the executive committee. Despite Robert Pollard's hope that euthanasia would receive such strong popular support that it would be debated in the House of Commons, Members of Parliament had been persistently unwilling to introduce the Bill and consequently the House of Lords was once again the forum for the debate. The Bill of 1969 differed considerably from its predecessor. It marked a notable shift in policy because for the first time it endorsed the notion of an advance declaration, which was said to accord with a 'deeply felt need'. The Society had received many letters from people reconciled to the fact that they had an incurable and progressive disease but who feared that their suffering might become unbearable. Letters had also come from individuals who had 'witnessed the pain, distress, and above all, the humiliation which, contrary to popular belief, are so often associated with a slow process of dying'. It was thought that the statutory declaration would reassure people that 'their expressed wish should command respect when the alternative to merciful release from illogical and intolerable suffering is a cruel deferment of inevitable death'. Indeed, it was considered by some to be a 'fundamental human right'.[77] The 'advance declaration' was regarded as a turning point in the 'furtherance of the Society's aims'. It would enable the Society's 'area of concern to extend to a patient who has become incapable of making a lucid decision, and also enables a patient to receive euthanasia without having to go through the much criticised deathbed formalities that have alienated half-committed sympathisers in the past'.[78]

The Bill entitled patients to euthanasia who at least thirty days previously had declared their wish for it. Two doctors, one of whom would need to be a consultant, would be required to certify that the patient was considered to be suffering 'from one of the "irremediable conditions" specified in article A, B or C of his declaration'. The important shift to note here is the substitution of 'irremediable conditions' for 'fatal illness accompanied by severe pain'. 'Irremediable condition' was defined as

(a) a condition of physical illness thought in the patient's case to be incurable and terminal and expected to cause him severe distress; or

(b) a condition of grievous physical affliction occasioning the patient serious injury or disability thought to be permanent and expected to cause him severe distress; or

(c) a condition of physical brain damage or deterioration such that the patient's normal mental faculties are severely and irreparably impaired.[79]

In the Bill's final draft, 'incapacity for rational existence' was added to 'expected to cause distress'. These changes expanded considerably the range of cases in which euthanasia might be performed. The Bill effectively enabled the individual to decide when his or her own life had ceased to be worthwhile; thereby endorsing a hedonistic preoccupation with quality of life.

The Bill of 1936 had tried to assist terminally ill patients suffering from severe pain, and to relieve the physician from the dilemma involved in administering successively larger doses of analgesic drugs which would accelerate his patient's death. In the thirty-three years since this issue had been discussed in the House of Lords, the view had been growing in influential circles that it was ethically justifiable to administer pain-killing drugs even though this might shorten life. Indeed, there was comparatively little debate about the ethical status of the doctrine of double effect; twenty-years previously this would have been controversial. The principle now seemed to be widely accepted.[80] The debate had shifted towards the wilful precipitation of death when life was considered not worthwhile whether death was imminent or not. The Bill of 1969 dealt with those cases where severe pain did not offer this increasingly acceptable ethical solution. As Lord Raglan, who introduced the Bill noted, the 'doctor's dilemma' arose 'principally where there is not the presence of great pain to provide an obvious guide as to what to do'.[81] The proposed reform would enable doctors to respect their patients' wishes. Medical science had enabled people to look forward to a longer span of life than ever before, but in keeping patients alive it also facilitated a 'twilight' existence between life and death. 'Their bodies and their personalities may have disintegrated to such a degree that life has become a meaningless burden to them and they look forward to the relief which death can bring them.'[82] Raglan saw the Voluntary Euthanasia Bill as a 'liberal and humanitarian measure for those who treasure for themselves the quality of life as much as its quantity'.[83]

In introducing the Bill to the Lords, Raglan, who was also a member of the National Secular Society, suggested that public opinion was inclining towards changing the law. He noted a trend towards legislation emphasising the 'freedom of the individual' which had been ably demonstrated by the Abortion Bill and the Suicide Bill.[84] The reform of euthanasia lagged behind suicide and abortion because of the nature of the interest group. '[T]hose who most wish for it, the old and the very infirm, are, by their very nature, not in a position to mount an energetic and articulate campaign.'[85] The Suicide Act had already granted citizens the right to kill themselves, and legalising voluntary euthanasia would merely extend the liberty 'under certain safeguards, to those dying people who are in no position to help themselves and would like to have their lives terminated by the kindly action of medication administered by the agency of another'.[86] Several other speakers said the same. The Earl of Listowel, the only member present in the House who had spoken in the debate of 1936 and voted for the first Voluntary Euthanasia Bill, saw the new Bill as a logical progression from the legalisation of suicide.[87] He thought the ethical case for voluntary euthanasia stronger than for suicide. Suicide was invariably the cowardly act of 'someone running away from responsibility'. Euthanasia on the other hand was likely to be the rational decision of someone whose life had become an intolerable burden to himself and others.

The debate was particularly interesting from a medical perspective. Raglan noted that while the British Medical Association vehemently opposed legalising voluntary euthanasia, many doctors favoured a highly paternalistic approach to their patients into which the law would have very little insight. It was noted that wealthier patients who had access to an understanding doctor in an accommodating nursing home found it easier to secure a good death than their poorer counterparts. Doctors in National Health hospitals had to follow very strict rules, and even if a particular doctor approved of euthanasia he risked being reported by those who did not. 'So, apart from the usual luck of the draw as who happens to be your doctor, what we have at the present time is a better opportunity for the rich than for the poor.'[88]

However, in January 1965 National Opinion Polls sampled 1,000 doctors, of whom 76.2 per cent agreed to the suggestion that 'some medical men do in fact help their patients over the last hurdle in order to save them unnecessary suffering, even if that involves some curtailment of life'.[89] No less than 36.4 per cent said they would administer voluntary euthanasia if it were legal. Far from undermining the doctor–patient relationship, Raglan claimed that it would be strengthened because the patient would know that the doctors, rather than keeping him alive as long as possible, would end life should it become unbearable.[90] Lord Platt, the only medical peer to speak in favour of the Bill, endorsed a number of these points. While noting that few people seemed to mind if the life of a terminally-ill patient was shortened by a few hours or days by pain-killing drugs, Platt sought to focus attention on what he considered the more pressing, yet contentious issue. He depicted the case of someone afflicted by a stroke 'paralysed in speech and limb' confined to bed for years, a perpetual burden to relatives and of use neither to themselves not society. While the Earl of Cork and Orrery had objected to the notion of an advance directive, it was precisely this aspect of the Bill which Lord Platt found most appealing.[91] Of course the Bill was not without significant opposition. As we have seen, the hospice movement had gone some way to diminishing the need for euthanasia. In the course of his introductory address Raglan conceded that hospices were a tremendous boon which made death comparatively comfortable, but because of their scarcity euthanasia was a necessity.

It might be said that if everyone could spend his last days in such surroundings there would be no need for this Bill. But not only would that leave out of the account the fact that, out of approximately 680,000 people who die in this country every year, only a fraction can go into such an institution – though with money and education that situation might in time be changed – it leaves out those who do not wish to eke out their lives in this way. Indeed, about half the 680,000 I have mentioned die in their home or a relative's home, and it seems very understandable that they should wish to. I myself should like to die in my own home if I could.[92]

Several peers seized upon these remarks, including Lord Thurlow, who also happened to be the chairman of St Christopher's Hospice. He suggested that rather than legalising euthanasia, more money should be devoted to geriatric units, hospices, research into pain relief, and adequate social services which would keep people 'active and happy in their own homes'. The House of Lords debate was to be welcomed because it underlined these needs, but he thought Raglan's solution misguided. It was an 'appalling confession of failure to admit, as I think he did, that we should legalise euthanasia because there are not enough places like St Christopher's'.[93] Lord Raglan protested rather unconvincingly that he had not made such a claim.

We should note, however, that a high proportion of the speeches made against the Bill centred upon more technical objections. Indeed the Earl of Cork and Orrery, who moved that the second reading of the Bill should be delayed for six months, based his speech on the supposition that it was simply a 'bad bill'. He was in a 'position of some strangeness' because he was urging the rejection of a Bill 'while approving, or at any rate sympathising with, its aims'.[94] He considered the Bill to have been drafted in a shoddy fashion with numerous loopholes, dangerous ambiguities and inadequate safeguards.[95] '"So far as we are aware", "the declarent appeared", "we believe" – how could you ever hope to pin anyone down on such negative non-committal testimony as that?'[96]

Alongside the objections to the specific clauses of the Bill, there were more profound objections. Lord Brock found the whole idea of euthanasia simply abhorrent. His reaction was 'one of extreme distaste and of some dismay that it should have been introduced'.[97] He also remarked that if society wished to 'destroy the sick' it should do so itself rather than getting the medical profession to act as executioner. Perhaps not surprisingly, bearing in mind that the prospective scope of patients to be included in the Bill had increased, the notion of a slippery slope reappeared. The Earl of Cork and Orrery foresaw the extension of euthanasia to the 'psychotic criminal' and non-voluntary euthanasia for the 'congenitally insane'. In his view these were progressions which seemed to lead inexorably to the excesses of 'Nazi Germany'.[98]

Lord Longford reinforced these sentiments, suggesting that the legalisation of voluntary euthanasia would lead to the introduction of compulsory euthanasia 'as sure as night follows day'. Having abandoned the concept of life being sacred there would be a tendency to enquire as to the value of the 'existence of X or Y', for example a 'defective child' or the elderly. Even if euthanasia were to remain strictly voluntary it would 'make suicide seem a natural course in many varied circumstances'. Pressures would be brought to bear on those who were making no obvious contribution to society. 'The question, "What is the use of me?" would begin to carry widespread terror especially among those with sensitive or scrupulous minds or delicate nerves or, for that matter, with unsympathetic relations'.[99] The slippery-slope argument was difficult to rebut. Not only because speakers persistently referred to the termination of the *non compos mentis*, but also because of the precedent set by the Abortion Law Reform Act of 1967 which had allegedly produced a situation in which a woman could have an abortion performed practically on demand.

Other peers seem to have been particularly attracted to the idea of non-voluntary euthanasia for the *non compos mentis*. The Earl of Huntingdon drew attention to the case of a teenage girl who had been involved in a car accident which left her brain 'completely destroyed' although her heart and lungs were in perfect health. The doctor observed that she might live anywhere between a few weeks and many years. 'But whatever happened her brain could never be restored, and all that could be offered to her was a life in bed and being artificially fed through her veins. That is the sort of case which makes us wonder about euthanasia.'[100] Lord Clifford of Chudleigh also felt that there were strong arguments for euthanasia.[101] His views on the subject had been reinforced by a visit to an old people's hospital where he had been struck by the sight of rows of beds 'each holding a human being lying inert, some sleeping, some perhaps under sedation, some with their eyes open looking utterly listless, hopeless, lifeless in a kind of torpor. One felt stifled with the all pervading apathy, the lethargy of the whole atmosphere, the intense sadness of the whole scene.'[102] Similarly the Bishop of Durham, while noting that the case for voluntary euthanasia seemed to have been weakened by developments in the pharmacological relief of pain, suggested, 'Something like euthanasia might well in principle be morally justified in the keeping alive of people by extraordinary means', particularly in cases of 'vegetative existence'.[103] These views were endorsed by Lord Longford, who directed attention to the sometimes officious approach of the medical profession which sought to preserve life without due regard for its quality, particularly brain-damaged patients who had no hope of regaining consciousness.[104] Lord Soper's view exemplifies the attitudes of a number of peers. He supported the idea of euthanasia and also thought it inappropriate to keep human vegetables alive:

> I am perfectly well persuaded that there are innumerable instances in the dark places of the hospital wards of animate yet not sentient creatures living an entirely vegetable existence – if, indeed, one can say that they are living at all ... surely it is rather silly to talk as if any organism which shows the outward and visible signs of sense reaction or of mechanical stimulation should be regarded as of sacred value.[105]

Despite this, he could not support the Bill because he considered it to have been ineptly drafted, as the Earl of Cork and Orrery had suggested.

Although the Bill was defeated, it was clear that a number of peers who had voted against the Bill had done so not because they were opposed to the principle of voluntary euthanasia but because they disliked certain details of the Bill. The Lords' debate had generated considerable publicity; all forms of media carried articles, letters and features on euthanasia and it seems fairly clear that increased support for euthanasia reflected the increased press coverage. The Secretary's report of 1969 gained confidence from the growing support within the 'younger generation'; there was a marked increase in requests for literature and speakers from 'individual students, schools, colleges and universities. An opinion poll of 2,000 young men and women, conducted by Mass Observation Limited, showed that 51 per cent agreed and only 28 per cent disagreed with voluntary euthanasia for those "incurable and in pain"'.[106] In 1970 it was noted that during the past year there had been 'growing recognition that major advances in the fields of medicine, science, surgery, biology and geriatrics pose tremendous medical and ethical problems'. Especially significant was an article published in the Catholic newspaper *The Tablet* on 28 June 1969, which suggested that the time had come 'to discuss in all seriousness the individual's right to life at any cost and his right to a dignified terminal illness and death, not hounded by doctors with a misguided sense of mission'.[107]

By the end of the 1960s discussion of euthanasia had become more intense than ever. The medical profession had hitherto been able studiously to avoid discussion of euthanasia, but in the new era of high-tech medicine, physicians had to concern themselves with the ethics of medical practice. Economic considerations reinforced the case for doing so. Although doctors could transplant hearts, it was very expensive to sustain the lives of the elderly, defective infants and human vegetables. Scarcity of resources required hard choices to be made.

Through the course of the 1960s medicine was able to save lives which would earlier have been lost. Yet there was considerable doubt about whether it was ethically and economically desirable to do. Such developments led the Euthanasia Society to broaden its proposals to include non-terminal cases. Because the medical profession had been forced to engage with these issues and because the public was increasingly exercised by the excesses of modern medicine, one might have assumed that euthanasia would have been legalised. Indeed, it seems fair to say that the Voluntary Euthanasia Bill of 1969 offered the best chance for success. But as we have seen, the attempt failed. In part the defeat can be attributed to the persistent objections which we have noted throughout preceding chapters. In particular the notion of a slippery slope seemed to have been reinforced by the Society's proposals for euthanasia in non-terminal cases and by the involvement of Society members in discussion of non-voluntary euthanasia for defective infants. We might note that at the annual general meeting of 1969 a resolution was passed 'that the name of the Society be changed to the ... Voluntary Euthanasia Legalisation Society'. The mover, a Mr J. Partington said that 'when asked "what does euthanasia mean?" he felt he had to start making excuses and explain that it concerned only those who sought release from prolonged suffering'.[108] But the Bill's defeat probably had more to do with the perceived inadequacies of its safeguards.

In addition a number of rhetorical devices had been developed to contest the need for euthanasia. The increasing acceptance of the doctrine of double effect meant that the actions of the physician at the deathbed scene were not eyed too closely. The notion of a distinction between acts and omissions on the part of the physician also enabled the acceleration of death without placing the physician in a moral dilemma. As Peter Singer has suggested, 'it cannot be said that when a doctor refrains from treating a patient, the patient's death is caused by "nature" rather than by the doctor'. Both the illness and the omission are part of 'the sum total of the conditions positive and negative taken together which is the full causal account of the death'.[109] Nevertheless, such a rhetorical device enabled the physician to condone the accelerated death of a patient without endorsing the notion of active euthanasia.

Notes

1   Trevor Fisher, 'Permissiveness and the politics of morality', *Contemporary Record*, Vol. 7, No. 1, Summer 1993, pp. 149–65; Arthur Marwick, *British Society Since 1945* (Harmondsworth, 1982); Arthur Marwick, *The Sixties* (Oxford, 1998).

2   See Frank Dawtry, 'The abolition of the death penalty in Britain', *British Journal of Criminology*, Vol. 6, Apr. 1966, pp. 183–92.

3   Brian P. Block and John Hostettler, *Hanging in the Balance: A History of the Abolition of Capital Punishment in Britain* (Winchester, 1997).

4   Barbara Brookes, *Abortion in Britain 1900–1967* (London, 1988).

5   CMAC/SA/VES/C.8 Minutes of the AGM, 28 May 1964.

6   *The Lancet*, 5 Aug. 1961, p. 305.

7   *Ibid.*, p. 306.

8   J. M. Hinton, 'The physical and mental distress of the dying', *Quarterly Journal of Medicine*, New Series 32, No. 125, Jan. 1963, pp. 1–21.

9   *Ibid.*, p. 15.

10   *Ibid.*, p. 20.
11   CMAC/SA/VES/B.12 The Voluntary Euthanasia Society, *The Case for Voluntary Euthanasia*, pp. 19–20.
12   Church of England Board for Social Responsibility, *On Dying Well: An Anglican Contribution to the Debate on Euthanasia* (London, 1976) p. 7.
13   *The Case for Voluntary Euthanasia*, p. 15.
14   P. I. Folb, *The Thalidomide Disaster and its Impact on Modern Medicine* (Cape Town, 1977) p. 3.
15   *Ibid.*, p. 4.
16   G. C. L. Bertram, 'The making and the taking of life: substance of a lecture to the Oxford Humanist Group, 5 Mar. 1963', *Eugenics Review*, Vol. 55, No. 3, Oct. 1963, pp. 159–65.
17   Reader's letter from G. Reichardt, *The Times*, 15 Nov. 1962, p. 13.
18   Reader's letter from Margery L. Spring Rice, *The Times*, 15 Nov. 1962, p. 13.
19   Reader's letter from I. B. G. Adaire, *The Times*, 19 Nov. 1962, p. 11.
20   CMAC/SA/VES/C.8 Euthanasia Society AR for 1962.
21   Bertram, 'The making and the taking', p. 164.
22   *Ibid.*, p. 163.
23   *Proceedings of the Royal Society of Medicine*, Vol. 60, Nov. 1967, Symposium on 'The cost of life', pp. 1195–246.
24   *Ibid.*, 1223.
25   R. B. Zachary, 'Ethical and social aspects of treatment of spina bifida', *The Lancet*, 3 Aug. 1968, p. 275.
26   Helga Kuhse and Peter Singer, *Should the Baby Live?* (Oxford, 1985) pp. 48–9.
27   Zachary, 'Ethical and social', p. 274.
28   *Ibid.*
29   See, 'New horizons in medical ethics', *BMJ*, 5 May 1973, pp. 284–9; 'Health Service or sickness service?', *BMJ*, 18 Dec. 1971, pp. 734–6.
30   Zachary, 'Ethical and social'.
31   Cited in Kuhse and Singer, *Should the Baby Live?*, p. 53.
32   See letter to the editor from Ian G. Wickes, 'Ethical and social aspects of treatment of spina bifida', The Lancet, 21 Sep. 1968, p. 677.
33   Walpole Lewin, Department of Neurological Surgery and Neurology, Addenbrooke's Hospital, Cambridge, and Army Neurosurgical Unit, Colchester, 'Severe head injuries', *Proceedings of the Royal Society of Medicine*, p. 1208.
34   *Ibid.*, pp. 1208–9.
35   *Ibid.*, p. 1209.
36   *The Lancet*, 8 Dec. 1962, p. 1205.
37   *Ibid.*
38   *Ibid.*
39   CMAC/SA/VES/C.8 Memorandum for AGM 1966, Agenda Clause 7 – Policy, proposed by C. E. Vulliamy.
40   *Proceedings of the Royal Society of Medicine*, p. 1216.
41   'The importance of death', *World Medicine*, 13 Aug. 1968, p. 24.
42   CMAC/SA/VES/o/s 1 *The Observer*, 29 Sep. 1967, p. 29.
43   *Old Age* (Office of Health Economics, London, 1968) p. 3.
44   'The importance of death', p. 28.
45   Professor Sir Denis Hill, Institute of Psychiatry, 'Economic and ethical considerations arising from modern care of the defective child and the very

old', *Proceedings of the Royal Society of Medicine*, p. 1233.
46 CMAC/SA/VES/b.9 *The Observer Review*, 24 Sep. 1967.
47 See *New Statesman*, 29 Sep. 1967, p. 399.
48 See for example *Freethinker*, Vol. 88 No. 4, 26 Jan. 1968, p. 25.
49 John Rowan Wilson, 'The freedom to die', *The Spectator*, 7 Feb. 1969, p. 169.
50 Donald Gould, 'The new doctor's dilemma', *New Statesman*, 29 Sep. 1967, p. 399.
51 CMAC/SA/VES/B.12 The Euthanasia Society Newsletter, No. 6, Nov. 1967.
52 CMAC/SA/VES/B.9 *The Observer Review*, 24 Sep. 1967.
53 *BMJ*, 17 Feb. 1968, p. 442.
54 *Ibid.*
55 *Ibid.*
56 CMAC/SA/VES/B.9 *The Observer Review*, 24 Sep. 1967.
57 Church of England Board for Social Responsibility, *Decisions About Life and Death: A Problem in Modern Medicine* (London, 1966) pp. 7–8.
58 *Ibid.*, p. 30.
59 *Ibid.*, p. 9.
60 *The Lancet*, 23 Oct. 1965, pp. 801–5.
61 *The Lancet*, 23 Oct. 1965, p. 803.
62 Roy Porter, *The Greatest Benefit to Mankind: A Medical History of Humanity from Antiquity to the Present* (London, 1997) pp. 684–7.
63 *Decisions About Life and Death*, Appendix 1, Some legal aspects of one's duty to the sick, by Chancellor E. Garth Moore, p. 43.
64 *Ibid.*, Appendix 1, pp. 46–7.
65 CMAC/SA/VES/C.8 Minutes of the AGM, 20 Dec. 1968.
66 CMAC/SA/VES/B.12 *The Euthanasia Society Newsletter*, No. 5, Jul. 1967.
67 *Ibid.*
68 *Ibid.*
69 CMAC/SA/VES/C.8 Secretary's report to the AGM 11 Dec. 1967.
70 CMAC/SA/VES/B.12 *The Euthanasia Society Newsletter*, No. 6, Nov. 1967.
71 *Ibid.*
72 CMAC/SA/VES/B.12 *The Euthanasia Society Newsletter*, No. 7, Jun. 1968, p. 3.
73 *Ibid.* pp. 4–5.
74 CMAC/SA/VES/C.8 Secretary's report to the AGM 20 Nov. 1968.
75 CMAC/SA/VES/o/s 1 *South London Press*, 9 Feb. 1968.
76 CMAC/SA/VES/o/s 1 *The Universe*, 29 Mar. 1968.
77 CMAC/SA/VES/C.8 Secretary's report to the AGM, 20 Nov. 1968.
78 *The Draft Bill*, p. 1.
79 *Ibid.*, pp. 5–6.
80 See Lord Longford's speech, Voluntary Euthanasia Bill, *H.L. Deb.* 25 Mar. 1969, c. 1190.
81 *Ibid.*, c. 1149.
82 *Ibid.*, cols 1145–6.
83 *Ibid.*, c. 1151.
84 *Ibid.*, c. 1144.
85 *Ibid.*
86 *Ibid.*, c. 1145.
87 *Ibid.*, c. 1211.
88 *Ibid.*, c. 1148.
89 *Ibid.*

90 *Ibid.*, c. 1151.
91 *Ibid.*, cols 1201–2.
92 *Ibid.*, c. 1146.
93 *Ibid.*, c. 1201.
94 *Ibid.*, c. 1151.
95 *Ibid.*, c. 1152.
96 *Ibid.*, c. 1154.
97 *Ibid.*, c. 1173.
98 *Ibid.*, c. 1159.
99 *Ibid.*, cols. 1192–4.
100 *Ibid.*, c. 1218.
101 *Ibid.*, c. 1207.
102 *Ibid.*, cols 1186–7.
103 *Ibid.*, c. 1180.
104 *Ibid.*, c. 1190.
105 *Ibid.*, c. 1196.
106 CMAC/SA/VES/C.8 Secretary's report to the AGM, 5 Nov. 1969.
107 CMAC/SA/VES/C.8 Secretary's report to the AGM, 30 Nov. 1970.
108 CMAC/SA/VES/C.8 Minutes of the AGM, 5 Nov. 1969.
109 Kuhse and Singer, *Should the Baby Live?*, p. 83.

Conclusion and epilogue

The modern euthanasia debate was begun in 1870 by amateur philosopher S. D. Williams jun., a member of the Birmingham Speculative Club. Precisely why the 1870s should have witnessed an intense, albeit short-lived, debate on mercy-killing is not immediately apparent. But a number of catalysts have presented themselves. To a certain degree, the debate can be seen as an offshoot of a pre-existing and broader debate on suicide as a whole. This debate had become particularly vibrant during the late eighteenth century following the publication of David Hume's essay *On Suicide*, in which he had argued that man had a 'native liberty' to choose the time of his own death. Significantly he had cited the specific circumstances of pain and disease. The arguments advanced in favour of euthanasia by authors such as Samuel Williams, Lionel Tollemache and Annie Besant betrayed the heavy influence of this work, especially with their attempts to demonstrate the alleged hypocrisy surrounding the Christian concept of the sanctity of human life. Developments in anaesthetics and palliative drugs had also made euthanasia an important issue of practical ethics at this time. The use of these drugs had itself been the subject of considerable controversy, being interpreted in some religious quarters as indicative of impatience with the ways of Providence. But not only did they offer a way of avoiding suffering, these drugs could also accelerate death. If this was considered legitimate, then the sanctity of human life, which was regarded as a concept which did not admit of degrees, was very difficult to sustain.

Since the time of St Thomas Aquinas, the belief that all forms of self-murder were a mortal sin had effectively precluded the practice of physician-assisted suicide. By drawing attention to shortcomings in the sanctity of human life as a coherent concept, the early euthanasiasts highlighted the need for alternative criteria upon which the worth of human life might be determined. This produced a variety of different arguments in favour of a variety of different types of euthanasia. The publication of Williams's essay also coincided with the decline of the evangelical movement replete with its distinct notion of the 'good death'; a notion in which spiritual well-being had primacy over physical well-being. Previously pain had been regarded as something to be borne with fortitude. The time was thus particularly propitious for a discussion of euthanasia.

By reconstructing the first euthanasia debate, we have resisted the temptation to project modern day notions of euthanasia onto previous epochs. Having examined precisely what was said and why, we have avoided the assumption that there is something time-less about euthanasia debates. By examining systematically all literature pertaining to euthanasia it has become clear that even after the emergence of the physician-assisted suicide notion of euthanasia, the term embraced a number of different meanings. The notion of the 'good death' could be construed in numerous different ways which in turn raised questions of a 'good death' for whom and from whose perspective.

We have seen that social Darwinian and eugenic thought were strong themes of the euthanasia debate. The perceived counter-selectivity of modern society, combined with heightened concerns about the incurability and apparent rising tide of lunacy and mental deficiency elicited proposals for the killing of defectives. This partic-ular interpretation of the 'good death' featured prominently in the first euthanasia debate and deserves a far more central position in the history of the British euthanasia movement than it has received hitherto.

Although our analysis of the first euthanasia debate has revealed a very rich discussion with several different notions of the good death – including requested mercy-killing in the specific circum-stances of incurable disease, altruistic suicide and the non-voluntary mercy-killing of the *non compos mentis* on alleged humanitarian, economic and eugenic grounds – it is also clear that the medical profession was not engaged in this debate during the nineteenth century. These discussions were primarily philosophical. Prior to the twentieth century, euthanasia in the mercy-killing sense failed to make any significant impact within the British medical profession. Suicide remained highly contentious, and it would have been rather unrealistic to have expected a medical profession, as conservative as Britain's was at this time, to have pioneered a proposal as radical as mercy-killing; a practice which was prohibited by its ethical code, by the law, and by the Christian concept of the sanctity of human life. However, the evidence suggests that perhaps the overriding reason why physicians were not occupied with euthanasia in the mercy-killing sense was because they were concerned with securing it in a more classical sense. Indeed the only medical text to use the term euthanasia in its title was a book by William Munk which was concerned with methods of making a patient comfortable during his last hours or days. Drugs might be used in this endeavour, but wilful precipitation of death was not the objective. Ironically, it was observed that the administration of palliative drugs frequently prolonged rather than shortened life. This interpretation contrasts sharply with previous accounts, which have suggested that after 1870 there was considerable discussion of the mercy-killing variety of euthanasia among physicians.

It was only at the turn of the century that an English doctor first advocated mercy-killing. This proposal was isolated and elicited no discernible support. In proposing such a practice, Dr C. E. Goddard, a public health official, drew attention to the growing incidence of cancer, which had allegedly increased the frequency of painful deaths. Inadequacies in palliative care were seen as a strong justification for mercy-killing. This was a distinctly practical proposal and was largely free from the philosophical discussion which had marked the debate of the 1870s. Importantly, however, Goddard's proposals were juxtaposed with proposals for the mercy-killing of the *non compos mentis*. At the turn of the century, concern over the failure of the asylum and psychiatry more broadly to address the problems of lunacy and mental deficiency had been instrumental in eliciting eugenic proposals which occasionally fed into discussion of mercy-killing. We should note that Goddard's proposals did not use the term euthanasia and it is probably for this reason that they have been neglected by other historians. As we have noted throughout this book, euthanasia is a particularly problematic term. The term has not necessarily denoted mercy-killing. Similarly, discussion of forms of mercy-killing which approximate modern-day concepts of euthanasia have not always used that term. It is perhaps the failure to acknowledge this which has accounted for the anaemia of previous studies.

For much of the late nineteenth century and the early twentieth century, discussion about euthanasia was decidedly fragmented, so much so, that it is hardly meaningful to speak of an organised euthanasia movement before the 1930s. Indeed, the few existing accounts which have looked at the British euthanasia movement depict a period of quietude from the early twentieth century until the 1930s. But this is a little simplistic. Discussion of mercy-killing did persist, although the term euthanasia was not always used. This discussion took place in a number of rather diverse publications and engaged authors drawn from the disparate fields of theology, philosophy and psychiatric medicine. During this period, euthanasia in the classical sense was almost entirely replaced by the concept of mercy-killing. But the concept continued to embrace two distinct meanings: mercy-killing for the *compos mentis*, and non-voluntary mercy-killing for the mentally defective. For much of the period it was the second of these two proposals which received most attention, although ultimately it was rejected.

By examining this disparate discussion we are able to identify important themes which remain pertinent to the following years; notably the discussion of mercy-killing for mental defectives. To some degree this was underwritten by crude economic arguments which sought to save on scarce public finances by dispensing with individuals who were regarded as less worthwhile than the mentally unimpaired. It was also believed that the life of the mental defective was of such poor quality that it was actually of negative value. In contrast to the *compos mentis* patient who would be the subject of voluntary euthanasia, the mental defective was incapable of requesting a premature death. For some, however, this was insufficient reason to deny him relief from his suffering. But not all proposals for non-voluntary mercy-killing were based upon such apparently humanitarian concerns. The benefits to be derived from non-voluntary mercy-killing were not seen as pertaining solely to the recipient. The practice was also seen as a mechanism for relieving relatives of a crippling burden. We have seen numerous allusions to the lives of healthy citizens being 'wasted' on caring for hopelessly defective offspring. The justification for non-voluntary euthanasia was also partly eugenic. Such ideas were to some extent a logical concomitant to the radicalisation of eugenic ideas which was in progress at this time. Modern warfare was perceived as having led to a dilution of racial vitality. Segregation, sterilisation and birth control were usually seen as the most effective and desir able way of limiting the number of defectives in society, but it would have been possible to effect such change via the death rate as well as the birth rate. We are thus presented with the paradoxical situation whereby human loss on an unprecedented scale seemed to make questions of mercy-killing rather peripheral, yet altered the ethical climate sufficiently to allow such issues to be discussed far more openly than before the war. This was a time at which contentious issues in the moral sphere such as contraception, eugenic sterilisation and divorce all gained some ground. In this climate we can identify a greater readiness to discuss euthanasia. We might note, however, that contrary to what is often assumed, proposals for voluntary mercy-killing during this period tended to be distilled from proposals for the non-voluntary mercy-killing of mental defectives. This is an interesting rejoinder to those who argue that voluntary euthanasia is the thin end of a wedge that will lead inexorably to non-voluntary euthanasia for the *non compos mentis*.

In the 1930s voluntary euthanasia became a practical proposal emanating from the medical profession, championed by a number of well-known progressive reformers from the field of public health. Among these, Charles Killick Millard and C. J. Bond were the most significant. In 1935 a Voluntary Euthanasia Legalisation Society was established which sought to secure legislative endorsement of euthanasia. Several members of the Society's consultative medical committee also served on the Ministry of Health cancer committee, and it was the increased incidence of this disease and subsequent painful deaths which was repeatedly cited as the reason why euthanasia should be legalised.

In addition to the medical component of the Society there were also a number of ecclesiastics. This would have been practically inconceivable in the late nineteenth century. But the Society seems to have been rather successful in combating theological opposition. In 1935 fifteen prominent church leaders signed a statement published by the Voluntary Euthanasia Legalisation Society proclaiming that in their opinion euthanasia was not contrary to the teachings of Christ. Nor were theological arguments the primary cause of the defeat of the Voluntary Euthanasia (Legalisation) Bill in 1936. Indeed, while the Archbishop of Canterbury felt unable to support the Bill, his opposition was not based on theological grounds. Yet, to conclude from this that it was the existence of the Society which had transformed attitudes is clearly a little deterministic. Indeed, it is rather difficult to establish the extent to which the Society has been instrumental or incidental in changing theological attitudes to euthanasia. Bearing in mind that the ethical statement was signed only a year after the foundation of the Society it seems rather far-fetched to suppose that the Society was responsible for effecting a change in the views of ecclesiastics who were overturning the centuries-old concept of the sanctity of human life. It seems more likely that changing attitudes to euthanasia have been merely one aspect of a broader shift in attitudes to a complex of social issues including contraception, abortion and divorce.

In accounting for the failure of the Voluntary Euthanasia (Legalisation) Bill of 1936, several factors have been highlighted. Previous accounts have singled out the speeches made against the Bill by two medical peers, Lord Dawson and Lord Horder, but this seems an inadequate explanation. As the Society would itself acknowledge, the legislation which it sought to introduce was a radical departure from custom and tradition. The Bill of 1936 was an opening shot by a Society which had been formed only a year earlier, and it would not have been realistic to expect a legislative victory at this early stage. Particularly difficult to overcome were objections concerning the change to the ethos of the physician which the Bill represented. The notion that the doctor should be an executioner as well as a healer was anathema to many. This was compounded by the uncertainty which was endemic to medical decision making; most notably the potential of terminal diagnoses being made inaccurately. But while medical voices were certainly raised in opposition to the Bill, this should not necessarily be interpreted as evidence of stern opposition to the practice of euthanasia. Indeed, there was considerable evidence of a paternalistic attitude prevailing among the medical profession. The impression given was that as the doctor knew precisely what to do and would not let his patient suffer excessively, the law should not concern itself with this most private of affairs between doctor and patient. The most striking illustration of this was that Lord Dawson, the King's physician who was the principal opponent of the Bill, was later revealed to have aided the death of George V with an injection of morphia.

Another important reason for the defeat of the Bill of 1936 was the prevalence of the slippery-slope argument. Repeatedly, it was suggested that the legalisation of voluntary euthanasia was a first step behind which lay the desire to extend mercy-killing to others, especially mental defectives. In part this was a device employed by opponents to worry the floating voter who was sympathetic to the more conservative proposal of voluntary euthanasia. However, on numerous occasions, influential figures within the euthanasia movement expressed sentiments which seemed to suggest that perhaps the legalisation of voluntary euthanasia was just a first step. This was the case with individuals such as C. J. Bond, the Chairman of the Voluntary Euthanasia Society, and R. F. Rattray, a signatory of the Society's ethical statement. Lord Ponsonby was another. While introducing the Voluntary Euthanasia (Legalisation) Bill to the House of Lords in 1936 Ponsonby remarked that 'we have restricted our proposals in this Bill purposely, whatever our views may be about Mongolians, congenital idiots and senile dementia, where safeguards would have to be very much more strict and where there would be no doubt other great difficulties'.[1]

The book has also revealed a largely neglected relationship between eugenics and euthanasia. Martin Pernick's observation that the terms euthanasia and eugenics are deeply value laden would seem to be a valid one. For as he suggests, euthanasia could mean judging who was better off dead, and eugenics could mean judging who was better not born. It is also true that both concepts have a history of overlap. But, this relationship needs to be treated carefully. It is inappropriate to suggest that all forms of non-voluntary euthanasia are eugenic. The primary motive prompting calls for the killing of mental defectives was humanitarian, they were underpinned by a desire to relieve suffering. All eugenic prescriptions were contentious, and euthanasia with a eugenic purpose was considered unacceptable and ineffective by all but the smallest minority. When Charles Killick Millard wrote to C. P. Blacker, the General Secretary of the Eugenics Society, it was recognised that only euthanasia for individuals who suffered from pronounced disability or deformity were of interest to the Eugenics Society. Even here, the eugenic bearing was thought to be small, as these individuals were never likely to become parents. While there has been a history of shared membership between the two Societies, we should note that membership of one Society did not dictate allegiance to the other. Lord Horder provides the classic example of this, for although he was a prominent eugenist, he opposed the Voluntary

Euthanasia (Legalisation) Bill in the Lords.

If a fusion of eugenics and euthanasia was not already politically undesirable enough, the revelations of the Nazi programme of non-voluntary euthanasia for defectives went some way to cementing this. Indeed, the British euthanasia movement could not avoid being tarred with the Nazi brush. This was particularly apparent during the House of Lords debate of 1950 when slippery-slope arguments were again very much to the fore. But perhaps rather surprisingly these revelations also elicited sympathetic proposals for the non-voluntary killing of defectives; proposals which would not have been out of place in Nazi Germany. Occasionally these remarks were made by such controversial and outspoken figures as Dr E. W. Barnes, the Bishop of Birmingham, but at other times by leading figures within the field of British psychiatry, notably A. F. Tredgold and R. J. A. Berry.

During the 1950s the fortunes of the British euthanasia movement experienced a sharp decline. The association of the term 'euthanasia' with Nazi atrocities was undoubtedly important, but so were internal changes which left the Society bereft of leadership. These problems were compounded by a seemingly conservative moral climate and a palliative care movement which appeared to be undermining the case for voluntary euthanasia.

During the 1960s the euthanasia movement enjoyed a reversal of fortunes. To some extent this was a function of internal factors, and a degree of consistency was restored to the leadership of the Society. But the moral climate was also far more propitious. This was a decade during which legislation and attitudes towards homosexuality, contraception, abortion, the death penalty and suicide were all liberalised. In addition, medical innovations such as the respirator, and medical disasters such as thalidomide had begun to raise profound questions about the prolongation of life when quality of life was clearly being supplanted by mere quantity. The euthanasia debate changed markedly during this period from a relatively straightforward concern with the relief of pain towards a preoccupation with an apparent conflict between patient autonomy and the actions of an overly officious medical profession. Precisely how influential the Voluntary Euthanasia Society had been in returning the issue to the practical agenda remains a little unclear. Certainly, members of the Society such as Glanville Williams, Eliot Slater and Leonard Colebrook were heavily involved in the debate.

But, it would appear that the developments in medical technology, which made the question of quality versus quantity of life so pertinent during this period, set the agenda of discussion rather autonomously. The discussion shifted further towards an everyday concern of practical, medical ethics. It was during this decade that euthanasia stood its strongest chance of being legalised. Yet the Voluntary Euthanasia Bill of 1969 was defeated.

In the thirty or so years that have elapsed since the defeat of the Voluntary Euthanasia Bill of 1969, euthanasia has remained illegal. At first glance it would seem difficult to dispute that the euthanasia movement has been an unmitigated failure. But, on reflection, this verdict is unduly harsh. Three broad categories should be considered: religious attitudes, the legal position and medical practice. All of these issues have been instrumental in ensuring the prohibition of euthanasia, but they are no longer so resolute as they once were. Indeed, it is suggested that there is now considerable latitude surrounding the question of euthanasia.

For centuries the Christian notion of the sanctity of human life provided a powerful argument against all forms of suicide. It is also clear that the supporters of euthanasia have devoted tremendous effort to combating religious opposition, and in this endeavour they have met with some success. Increasingly it has become apparent that support for euthanasia and Christianity are not mutually exclusive. Of course religious opposition has not been silenced. Opposition on theological grounds has been voiced during every Parliamentary discussion of euthanasia. Throughout the study we have also seen that some of the most sustained opposition to euthanasia has been voiced in the Catholic press; notably *The Universe*, the *Catholic Herald* and *The Tablet*. These publications have been forthright in defending the position of St Thomas Aquinas concerning the sinfulness of suicide. But even the Catholic stance has not remained unaltered. In 1957, for example, the Pope granted cautious support to the doctrine of double effect; acknowledging that a doctor may administer successively larger doses of narcotic drugs to a patient if his intention is the relief of pain even though this might have the unintended consequence of shortening his patient's life. It seems clear that the sanctity of human life is no longer such a powerful obstacle to the euthanasia campaign as it once was. In 1993 an opinion poll conducted by National Opinion Polls for the Voluntary Euthanasia Society indicated a high level of support for voluntary euthanasia among all religious denominations. The question was rather ambiguous because it merely enquired whether the law should allow a patient suffering from an 'incurable physical illness' to receive 'medical help to a peaceful death'.[2] Nevertheless, the question was answered in the affirmative by 85 per cent of those who were members of the Church of Scotland, 80 per cent of Anglicans, 73 per cent of Roman Catholics, 60 per cent of Jews and 93 per cent of agnostics.[3] In the late twentieth century euthanasia became primarily a medico-legal problem rather than a theological one.

In 1870 when Samuel Williams advanced his argument in favour of euthanasia he did so partly because the case was easier to sustain than the case for suicide as a whole. Because suicide was often regarded as a cowardly act, euthanasia was depicted as a case apart. It was argued that a painful and terminal illness provided perhaps the most justifiable grounds for self-destruction. However, suicide as a whole has now been legalised. Supporters of euthanasia at the end of the nineteenth century would have seen this as a great triumph. We might also note that both the Church Assembly Board for Social Responsibility and a joint council of the British Medical Association and the Magistrates Association supported the decriminalisation of suicide and attempted suicide.[4] Paradoxically while suicide has been legalised, euthanasia has not. The reason for this apparent anomaly has been the alleged potential for abuse. During the suicide debate of 1961 the Lord Chancellor conceded that the 'moral culpability' of assisting suicide varied greatly.[5] The most acceptable case was that in which an individual provided drugs to a patient suffering from a 'painful and incurable illness' at their request. Indeed several speakers noted that the case for legalising mercy-killing was particularly strong. At the other end of the spectrum, however, was the person who aided or advised another's suicide for his own financial advantage. This led the Lord Chancellor to conclude that even when it was decided that 'the motives of a person who seeks to take his own life should no longer be the concern of the criminal law', the same could not be said 'of those who are involved in bringing about the death of another'.[6] As Lord Denning noted, this produced the rather strange situation whereby it became a criminal offence to aid, abet or procure an act which was not itself illegal.[7] To some extent the Suicide Act of 1961 must be seen as a success for the supporters of euthanasia. The Act removed the legal and moral censure of a terminally-ill patient who decided to take his own life. But for those patients who wished to die but were incapacitated and unable to effect their own death the Bill was of little practical help. The resulting legal position was such that a physician found to have assisted a suicide by placing lethal drugs in the hands of a patient would be liable to a period of imprisonment of up to fourteen years if convicted. If the doctor was found to have administered a lethal injection he could be charged with murder. But even from a legal perspective the question of euthanasia tends to be treated rather liberally. Such an interpretation is underlined by an examination of the history of the British euthanasia movement after 1969.

Following the defeat of Lord Raglan's Bill the Voluntary Euthanasia Society continued to receive strong support. Publicity for euthanasia continued to increase and so did membership of the Society; by 1971 there were over 800 members. But after another legislative defeat it was unclear what policy should be pursued. For a while the Society thought about resurrecting the idea of an amendment to the Suicide Act of 1961, but was unable to find an MP willing to sponsor such a measure. In 1973 a rather despondent Eliot Slater noted that the prospects of legislative success were slim. In place of another Voluntary Euthanasia Bill he thought it might be more profitable to act as a 'Right to Die' Society, encouraging the medical profession to be more responsive to patients' desires. This seemed to indicate that there was considerable scope for securing acceptable practice within the existing law. This view was reinforced by the Church of England, whose report on euthanasia noted that it was consistent to argue that euthanasia was morally permissible in certain cases but to oppose any change to the law. Legal reform might in practice lead to cases of euthanasia which should not be permitted. The law was considered to be a 'blunt instrument for dealing with moral complexities' and it was 'better to allow hard cases to be taken care of by the various expedients that are available than to introduce a new principle which would turn out to be too permissive'.[8] Despite such sentiment the Society eventually decided that another parliamentary Bill was appropriate.

In 1976 the Incurable Patients Bill was introduced to the House of Lords by Baroness Wootton of Abinger. The Bill had three main proposals. The first was that an incurable patient should be entitled to receive 'whatever quantity of drugs may be required to give him full relief from pain and physical distress, and to be rendered unconscious if no other treatment is effective to give such relief'. Secondly, an incurable patient who caused his own death by taking an overdose or any 'other intentional action' would be 'deemed to have died by misadventure'. No person would be 'under a duty to interfere with any course of action taken by an incurable patient to relieve his suffering in a manner likely to cause his own death, and any interference intentionally undertaken contrary to the known wishes of the patient shall be unlawful'. Finally, a patient who as a result of brain damage or degeneration became 'permanently incapable of giving directions' would 'be regarded as refusing to receive life sustaining treatment' if 'at an earlier date, when of sound mind', they had 'made an existing written statement attested by two witnesses declaring that in the event of his becoming so incapable he wishes not to receive such treatment'.[9] The word 'euthanasia' was studiously avoided. As Lord Raglan noted, the term had 'acquired some unfortunate connotations'. In many people's minds it had come to mean 'bumping off in a painless way someone who [was] not particularly wanted'. Raglan had been told by numerous people that they agreed that 'handicapped children' should not be allowed to 'survive'.[10]

The Bill was defeated by 85 votes to 23. The main reason for the defeat was that for many it seemed to serve no useful purpose. As Lord Wells-Pestell noted, the clause requiring the physician to provide his patient with sufficient drugs to ensure complete relief from physical pain and distress, did no more than reflect what he and many others considered to be 'existing good medical practice'. Doctors already had a professional duty to control pain to the best of their ability 'even in those cases where such a measure may hasten death'.[11] Indeed, Lord Dawson, a vehement opponent of legalising euthanasia had made precisely the same point in the House of Lords in 1936. During the 1930s Charles Killick Millard had argued that by administering successively larger doses of palliative drugs the doctor was hovering on the brink of manslaughter, but by the 1970s the legitimacy of double-effect was considered contentious by very few. Indeed the Crown Prosecution Service has stated explicitly that the actions of a doctor are lawful if, in the best interests of a terminally-ill patient, he administers pain-killing drugs even though the patient will probably die as a result. The Home Office has suggested that in this type of situation a criminal act may be committed, but this would depend on the intention of the doctor and whether it could be shown that his actions directly caused the patient's death. They emphasised that treatment administered 'should be necessary to the relief of pain'. Actions which had 'no pain-relieving qualities' but merely accelerated death were considered unlawful. It was also noted that the existing law was 'by and large, producing the right outcomes and not causing problems'.[12] But new complexities had been introduced into the euthanasia debate and particular aspects of the Incurable Patients Bill differed markedly from earlier attempts to legalise euthanasia. These concerned the futile prolonging of life and burdensome medical treatments; problems which were the product of the medical innovations of the 1950s and 60s. These concerns did not and could not have occupied the supporters of euthanasia before the late 1950s. Yet even with regard to these issues the medical profession had begun to assume a more flexible position. As Lord Wells-Pestell observed, 'any conscious, sane patient' was 'entitled to refuse any item of treatment to which he objects'.[13] In fact both of these points had been established in 1970 in the course of two meetings between representatives of the Voluntary Euthanasia Society and the Working Party of the British Medical Association's Board of Education and Science. At this time it had been established that a patient was entitled to refuse resuscitation in advance.[14] There had also been cautious support for allowing patients to die rather than striving officiously to keep them alive. When Eliot Slater had drawn attention to cases of advanced senility in which measures were taken to prolong life, the reply had been that there was no ethical or legal requirement to do so. 'The view seemed to be that it was alright to let them die by an act of omission but entirely wrong to bring about death by an act of commission'.[15] These views were reinforced by an article published in *Criminal Law Review* in 1976, which argued that 'the right of a patient to refuse treatment was clear in the law, but was frequently over-ridden'.[16]

In March 1978 the Secretary of the Voluntary Euthanasia Society, C. R. Sweetingham, decided to retire, having held the position for the previous fourteen years. He was replaced by Nicholas Reed the Assistant Secretary. The appointment of Reed ushered in a phase of radicalism seemingly engendered by a sense of frustration. The first sign of this radicalism was the Society's decision to publish a booklet entitled the *Guide to Self-Deliverance* which instructed readers in the most effective methods of killing themselves. The Annual General Meeting of 1979 approved the publication of the booklet by 155 votes to 11 and also voted to change the name of the Society to EXIT. This had been suggested by Eliot Slater, who thought it would bring the society in line with the American movement, and was not tainted by association with Nazi practices. The decision to publish the booklet was contentious, and while the committee was seeking legal advice Mrs Jean Davies introduced a motion of no confidence in the committee on account of their reticence about publishing the booklet. The whole committee was forced to stand for re-election. Maurice Millard, Miss Barrington and Miss Blackett all lost their seats. The Society thus had a new and militant committee. Following this, a member of the Society, Dr Scott, took out an injunction against the Society to prevent publication, but the booklet was eventually made available to those aged twenty-five or over who had been members of the Society for over three months.

In April 1982 the Attorney General demanded that the Society stop the distribution of the booklet and destroy all remaining copies because it was seen to contravene section two of the Suicide Act of 1961. The Society decided to contest the action and in 1983 won a victory of sorts when the Attorney General was refused the declaration he sought. However, Mr Justice Woolf made clear that by knowingly supplying the booklet to someone who intended to commit suicide the Society was exposing itself to the risk of prosecution. If the booklet were on general sale it was suggested, the risk of criminality would be smaller because the supplier would have no knowledge of the purchaser's intentions. The Society came to the conclusion that 'it would be inadvisable to resume distribution of the Guide'.[17]

The limits of the law regarding assisted suicide and homicide were also being put to the test in other ways at this time. In 1979 Colin Brewer, a former GP, published an article in which he admitted attempting to kill a patient suffering from terminal cancer by administering a lethal dose. The case was investigated by the Director of Public Prosecutions (DPP) but no prosecution was launched. It was suggested that the available evidence fell 'below the minimum necessary to support prosecution'.[18] According to the doctor, however, 'perfectly adequate evidence would probably have been available if anyone had wanted to collect it'.[19] A few months earlier, in a book entitled *Jean's Way*,[20] journalist Derek Humphry had admitted administering a lethal dose to his wife who was dying from breast cancer. The DPP had also decided not to prosecute this case. According to Brewer, the decision to prosecute neither Humphry nor himself citing 'insufficient evidence' as the reason, suggested 'a form of words designed to conceal the fact that policy in these matters is not to institute proceedings for euthanasia in the case of terminally ill patients who are in severe pain, especially if the drugs used are those commonly prescribed for sedation or analgesia'.[21] In both cases, it seems that the doctrine of double effect may have precluded a clear-cut prosecution even if there had been the will to pursue the matter.

The frustration which had become evident in the euthanasia movement reached its apogee in 1980 when Nicholas Reed the Secretary of the Society was charged with conspiring to aid suicide along with Mark Lyons, a member of the Society, who was also charged with murder and aiding a number of suicides. The DPP rosecutions did not claim that any of the deceased had been killed involuntarily and admitted that their cases were 'sad and in some cases heartrending'.[22] Both Reed and Lyons were convicted. Reed was sentenced to two and a half years' imprisonment having been found guilty on four charges. Mark Lyons was acquitted of murder but convicted on six others charges. He had spent a year on remand and was released with a two-year suspended sentence. One is naturally curious to know why Reed and Lyons had been prosecuted when Humphry and Brewer were not. Evidence aside, the DPP had little option but to make a distinction between the exceptional and compassionate actions of Humphry and Brewer on the one hand and the decision wilfully to flout the law by individuals committed to a cause.

EXIT noted that the case had been a 'serious blow'. It re-stated its purpose as having been to influence public opinion and bring about legislative reform so that the incurably ill would be 'entitled to medical help' to an 'easy death'. It was suggested that the Society did not, nor had it ever sought to 'provide a counselling service for individuals who wish to end their own lives, let alone to break the existing law by giving them practical assistance'.[23] The actions of Reed had been in direct contravention of the Society's stated aims and had been conducted without the knowledge of the committee. They had portrayed the Society in a very 'unfortunate light'. An editorial in the *Times Health Supplement* observed that although after forty years the Society had been comparatively successful in convincing the general public and the media of the case for voluntary euthanasia, it had achieved 'no success in Parliament or the legal and medical establishments'. The article suggested that in these circumstances it was not overly surprising that 'during the late 1970s the more militant members began to lose patience'.[24] At the Society's Annual General Meeting on November 1982 the Society voted by 1301 votes to 276 to change its name back to the Voluntary Euthanasia Society. The name EXIT had become too closely associated with the Reed/Lyons debacle. In the course of 1983 Lord Listowel accepted an invitation to resume the presidency of the Society.

In 1985 Lord Jenkins of Putney, a Vice-President of the Voluntary Euthanasia Society, attempted to amend the Suicide Act of 1961. His motion sought to allow an individual to use as a defence under the Act the claim that they acted 'on behalf of the person who committed suicide and in so acting behaved reasonably and with compassion and in good faith'.[25] The Bill, which was defeated by forty-eight votes to fifteen, did not attempt to remove the offence. This modest approach had been adopted in order to avoid placing the burden of executioner upon the doctor as the previous Voluntary Euthanasia Bills had done. The previous approach had elicited particularly strong opposition from the medical profession. The amendment was opposed on familiar grounds, namely the possibility of abuse. Although the term was not used, it is clear that Lord Jenkins had introduced his amendment in order to deal with a situation where euthanasia might be at issue. However, as numerous speakers suggested, existing law seemed to deal with such cases adequately. In order to prosecute a case of this nature the consent of the DPP would be required. Lord Denning suggested that in the 'ordinary case of mercy killing' the DPP should not and probably would not prosecute. In the past this had been less certain, as prosecutions were launched by the chief constable or the police. Lord Denning hoped and anticipated that a policy would evolve whereby cases in which someone had assisted the suicide of a severely ill patient would not be prosecuted. '[I]n a sense, without any amendment ... by this almost procedural means we can achieve the result which is desired.'[26] Lord Glenarthur added weight to this view by noting that between 1980 and 1984 there had been only ten convictions under the Suicide Act. As he suggested, the 'noble Lord's target' was therefore very narrow indeed'.[27] Thus, despite the remarks of the *Times Health Supplement* it would seem that a modicum of success had been achieved with regard to the position of the 'legal establishment'. Euthanasia had not been legalised, but there was some understanding that it should be dealt with sympathetically and leniently within the existing law.

The flexibility of the law has been mirrored to some extent by the stance adopted by the medical profession. In 1987 the British Medical Association established a working party to address the problem of euthanasia in response to a resolution passed at the Annual Representatives Meeting of the Association in 1986.[28] Although the report reiterated that it was ethically and legally unacceptable for a doctor to actively kill a patient, on a number of closely related issues there was considerable latitude. It was noted that the ability of modern medicine to 'prolong' and 'rescue' life was in tension with the increasingly prevalent notion of patient autonomy, 'a growing awareness of the rights of patients to make decisions about what shall and what shall not be done to them'.[29] Even though the report conceded that doctors might sometimes override the wishes of a patient – a form of medical paternalism – they did so only when there was reason to believe that a patient was not 'acting in accordance with reason'.[30] As we have noted, considerable concern had been voiced about the wanton use of 'high-technology medicine' during the 1960s. Many patients made it known that they had enjoyed a 'good life' and did not wish to be 'subjected to repeated heroic attempts to keep them alive'.[31]

Patients also expressed fears about being put on a respirator in order to sustain them 'for long periods while their life ebbs away'. But the BMA's report suggested that apparatus such as respirator support should be employed only so that patients might 'return to sentient life or remain capable of sentience'. There was no reason to 'prolong a respirator-dependent life in a patient who no longer has any prospect of appreciating the extension of "life"'.[32] There were, however, certain reservations. It was suggested that the withdrawal of 'nutrition and good nursing', was in a different class to the discontinuation of futile medical treatments.[33] Yet even here a qualification was made. Naso-gastric feeding or gastrostomy was said to constitute a medical intervention. It was justified only when it made 'possible a decent life in which the patient can reasonably be thought to have a continued interest'.[34] Many patients regarded such treatment with the same 'horror' as resuscitation and artificial ventilation, they were at liberty to request that particular forms of treatment should not be pursued. It was considered perfectly acceptable to discontinue hopeless treatment which served merely to prolong a patient's suffering. It was similarly legitimate to embark upon a course of treatment with the intention of relieving pain even though this might carry the risk of death. This was considered to be 'clearly different from intervening at a patient's request with the intention of ending their life'.[35] Intent was repeatedly stressed as the key concept. Although the report sought to make a strong distinction between active and passive measures on the part of a doctor, one might wish to distinguish between the official position of a professional body and the attitudes of individual doctors. In 1994 a poll of 273 doctors observed that 32 per cent of those who had been asked to take 'active steps' to hasten the death of a patient had done so. Some 46 per cent of respondents would have considered such action if it were legal.[36] A confidential survey of general practitioners indicated that almost half of those who replied admitted easing a patient's death.[37] 'Easing a patient's death' may of course be interpreted far more conservatively than meaning the application of active euthanasia, but taken together these poll results suggest that hastening the death of a patient is no longer anathema to many doctors.

Since 1992 the British Medical Association has publicly endorsed the principle of advanced directives 'as a method of expanding patient choice beyond the onset of mental incapacity'.[38] It has also supported the idea of a Health Care Proxy nominated by a patient to make decisions about treatment in the event that they should become unable to do so themselves. In contrast to its position as outlined in 1987 the British Medical Association now considers it 'unethical to carry out any medical procedure intended to benefit a patient when that person has indicated a competent refusal'. Indeed, 'depending on the circumstances such an action may also constitute an assault in law'. In 1993 Lord Allen of Abbeydale presented the Medical Treatment (Advance Directives) Bill, supported by the Voluntary Euthanasia Society, to the House of Lords, which sought to secure legislative recognition of advance directives and Health Care Proxies.[39] The Society hoped that the House of Lords' Select Committee which followed would propose a statute law securing the legal status of advance directives and 'protecting health care teams from fear of prosecution if they allow patient to die by respecting an advance directive's refusal of treatment'. Such a recommendation was not forthcoming. The reason for this, as in the case of the Incurable Patients Bill of 1976 and the Suicide Amendment Act of 1985 appears to have been because it was considered unnecessary. The Select Committee suggested that increasingly doctors realised that they were ethically obliged to 'comply with advance directives'. This was underlined by developments in case law. The conclusion of the Select Committee seemed to be that the forms were already binding.[40]

The House of Lords Select Committee on Medical Ethics acknowledged that there were particular cases where euthanasia might seem appropriate, but suggested that 'individual cases could not reasonably establish the foundation of a policy which would have such serious and widespread repercussions'.[41] Throughout the history of the British euthanasia movement a strong objection to legalising voluntary euthanasia has been the view that vulnerable individuals might feel pressured to request it. This concern was reiterated by the House of Lords Select Committee. The Lords also concluded that it was not possible to set safe limits on voluntary euthanasia. It was suggested that 'issues of life and death' did not 'lend themselves to clear definition', and consequently 'it would not be possible to frame adequate safeguards against non-voluntary euthanasia if voluntary euthanasia were legalised'. It was thought that liberalisation of the law would almost certainly lead to abuse. The dangers of decriminalisation were considered to outweigh the problems which it sought to address.[42] The fear of a slippery slope, an argument which has been such a feature of the euthanasia since its inception, was raised yet again. Ironically, it seems difficult to dispute that a considerable amount of non-voluntary euthanasia, albeit passive, is already practised and condoned by both the legal and medical establishments.

As noted in the previous chapter, the active treatment of spina bifida babies which had become standard practice in the 1960s was subjected to strong criticism. John Lorber, one of the pioneers of this treatment, reversed his initial enthusiasm and switched to a policy of selective non-treatment having observed that 'massive effort' had 'led to much avoidable suffering'.[43] Selective non-treatment is now widely endorsed. Indeed, the British Medical Association notes that 'a careful and sensitive view must be taken in this area of practice and that the overriding concern should be to relieve the distress of an afflicted infant'.[44] Its report of 1988 acknowledged that while some doctors believed that spina bifida babies should not be 'encouraged to die' and should receive all available treatment in order to allow the baby to 'develop its full potential', this was 'countered, to a certain extent, by a careful consideration of the harm that many such infants do to the families into which they are born, and the often blighted and miserable lives which they live'. Not only does this endorse a form of non-voluntary passive euthanasia, but it is justified in part by the interests of a third party, namely the parents. This view advanced by the official body of the British medical profession differs little from the proposals of C. J. Bond and R. F. Rattray; proposals which Charles Killick Millard had tried so hard to exorcise from the British euthanasia movement. Indeed the advocates of voluntary euthanasia have been attacked repeatedly because of an alleged desire to extend euthanasia to defective babies once voluntary euthanasia has been legalised. Paradoxically, precisely these cases now seem to be legitimate while voluntary euthanasia remains illegal.

With regard to non-voluntary euthanasia, one must also note the case of Tony Bland. Bland, a victim of the Hillsborough stadium disaster who, while not terminally ill, was left in a persistent vegetative state. He had no discernible level of consciousness and no prospect of recovery, but he was kept alive by means of artificial feeding. His parents and doctors were agreed that it was futile to keep him alive indefinitely. But when the doctor informed the coroner that he intended to withdraw artificial feeding he was warned that he might face prosecution. A complex legal case ensued in which the House of Lords was finally required to deliberate. The Lords agreed that feeding could be withdrawn. In so doing it was clear that a decision had been made that Tony Bland's life should be ended. In their view, withdrawal of artificial feeding could be seen as an omission and not as a deliberate killing. 'The question arose whether nutrition and hydration, when given by some invasive method ... should be regarded as form of medical treatment which could, like other forms of medical treatment, be discontinued if they appeared to be of no benefit to the patient. The courts decided that they should be so regarded'.[45] Lord Browne-Wilkinson hinted at the legal perversity whereby it was 'lawful to allow a patient to die slowly, although painlessly over a period of weeks from lack of food but unlawful to produce his immediate death by lethal injection'.[46] The British Medical Association considered that 'under certain strictly defined circumstances', it was 'ethically acceptable to withdraw artificial nutrition and hydration from patients' who had lost 'specific and definable neurological pathways, the result of which is the permanent loss of sensitivity to external stimuli and loss of sentience'.[47] Several bodies have dissented from this view. The Royal College of Nursing believed that to withdraw feeding and fluids was a different issue from the decision to curtail other medical interventions.[48] Healthcare Opposed to Euthanasia (HOPE) suggested that the Bland case signified a softening in the law towards intentional killing. Indeed, it remarked that legislation was perhaps necessary in order to 'reaffirm the previous prohibition of intentional killing, whether by act or omission'.[49] Bishop Christopher Budd and Archbishop Thomas Winning considered the decision in the Bland case to amount to 'intentional killing by starvation'.[50]

At the present time the press has drawn attention to a rather more insidious form of euthanasia. On 6 January 1999 *The Times* reported that the police and health officials were investigating the deaths of at least fifty hospital patients 'amid allegations of a creeping tide of backdoor euthanasia'.[51] Claims were being investigated that intravenous drips had been withheld from dehydrated patients 'often while they were under sedation, and left them to die from thirst'.[52] The majority of patients involved were thought to be sufferering from 'strokes, asthma, other common medical conditions and dementia'.[53] Some five hospitals in Surrey, Derby, Kent and Sussex were being investigated after complaints from relatives and nurses. The Crown Prosecution Service is currently considering whether to prosecute a case centring around the Kingsway Hospital in Derby where nurses suggested that sufferers from dementia on a psycho-geriatric ward were 'starved and dehydrated until they became so weak that they died from infections'.[54]

The views, policies and practices reviewed in this study seem to lend considerable support to the views of bio-ethicists Helga Kuhse and Peter Singer who have observed that with the exception of certain religious devotees 'no one really believes that all human life is of equal value'. Despite this, 'many people pay lip-service to this belief' and use various disguises to mask the hypocrisy of their actions. Other individuals while acknowledging that all human life is not of equal worth are unwilling to extinguish promptly a life which is no longer worth living. 'They too are trying to draw a veil over the extent to which their policies and practices are incompatible with the traditional Judaeo-Christian doctrine of the sanctity of human life.'[55]

Notes

1   *H.L. Deb.* 1 Dec. 1936, c. 469.
2   'More Britons say "Give us the right to die"', *Voluntary Euthanasia Society leaflet*, 26 Apr. 1993.
3   *Ibid.*
4   *H.L. Deb.* 2 Mar. 1961, Suicide Bill c. 249.
5   *Ibid.*, c. 250.
6   *Ibid.*
7   *Ibid.*, c. 265.
8   Church of England Board for Social Responsibility *On Dying Well: An Anglican Contribution to the Debate on Euthanasia* (London, 1975) p. 12.
9   Incurable Patients Bill, 12 Feb. 1976.
10   *H.L. Deb.* 12 Feb. 1976, c. 240.
11   *Ibid.*, c. 226.
12   *Report of the House of Lords Select Committee on Medical Ethics* (London, 1994) p. 20.
13   *H.L. Deb.* 17 Feb. 1976, c. 226.
14   CMAC/SA/VES/C.8 Secretary's report of meeting on 8 April with Working Party on Euthanasia set up by the BMA Board of Education and Science.
15   CMAC/SA/VES/C.8 Meeting with BMA, 5 Oct. 1970. Notes compiled by Secretary after telephone conversation with Dr Slater.
16   Ian Kennedy, 'The legal effect of requests by the terminally ill and aged not to receive further treatment from doctors', Criminal *Law Review*, 1976, pp. 217–32.
17   'The guide which way now?' Voluntary Euthanasia Society Newsletter, *No. 19, Sep. 1983*.
18   Colin Brewer, '"Insufficient evidence" – or a subtle shift in policy on euthanasia?', *World Medicine*, 13 Jan. 1979, p. 30.
19   *Ibid.*
20   Derek Humphry, *Jean's Way* (London, 1978).
21   Brewer, 'Insufficient evidence', p. 30.
22   *Exit News*, No. 12, Spring 1981.
23   *Ibid.*
24   Cited in *Exit News*, No. 12, Spring 1981.
25   *H.L. Deb.* 11 Dec 1985, Suicide Act 1961 (Amendment) Bill, c. 289.
26   *Ibid.*, cols 299–300.
27   *Ibid.*, c. 311.
28   *Euthanasia: Report of the Working Party to Review the British Medical Association's Guidance on Euthanasia* (London, 1988) p. 1.

29 *Ibid.*, p. 3.
30 *Ibid.*, p. 17.
31 *Ibid.*, p. 21.
32 *Ibid.*
33 *Ibid.*, p. 22.
34 *Ibid.*, p. 23.
35 *Ibid.*, p. 25.
36 B. J. Ward and P. A. Tate, 'Attitudes among NHS doctors to request for euthanasia', *BMJ*, Vol. 308, 21 May 1994, pp. 1332–4.
37 *Pulse*, Vol. 57, No. 43, 1 Nov. 1997, p.1.
38 British Medical Association Information Pack on Euthanasia (1998), BMA House, Tavistock Square, London.
39 *Voluntary Euthanasia Society Newsletter*, No. 48, Apr. 1993.
40 *Voluntary Euthanasia Society Newsletter*, No. 51, Apr. 1994.
41 *Report of the House of Lords Select Committee*, p. 48.
42 *Ibid.*, p. 49.
43 J. Lorber, 'Results of treatment of myelomeningocele', *Developmental Medicine and Child Neurology*, Vol. 13, 1971, p. 279.
44 *Euthanasia: Report of the Working Party BMA*, p. 36.
45 *Report of the House of Lords Select Committee*, p. 17.
46 *BMA Information Pack* (1988).
47 *Ibid.*
48 *House of Lords Select Committee*, p. 18.
49 *Ibid.*
50 *Ibid.*
51 'Police check hospitals over "backdoor euthanasia"', *The Times*, 6 Jan. 1999, p. 1.
52 *Ibid.*
53 *Ibid.*
54 *Ibid.*
55 Helga Kuhse and Peter Singer, *Should the Baby Live?* (Oxford, 1984) p. 96.

Select bibliography

Primary sources

Archives

Contemporary Medical Archives Centre, Wellcome Institute for the History of Medicine, London: Voluntary Euthanasia Society Papers; Eugenics Society Papers.
Public Record Office, Kew: Ministry of Health, and Foreign Office Papers.
Wellcome Unit for the History of Medicine Oxford: C. P. Blacker Papers.

Official publications

Mental Deficiency Act 1913. Suggestions and plans relating to the arrangements of institutions for defectives (Board of Control, London, 1919).
Report of the House of Lords Select Committee on Medical Ethics (London, 1994).
Report of the Interdepartmental Committee on Mental Deficiency 1925–29 (Wood Report) 3 vols. (1929).

Periodical and annual publications

House of Lords Debates.
Board of Control Annual Reports.
Annual Reports of the Chief Medical Officer of the Ministry of Health.

Books and articles

Bacon, Francis, *New Atlantis* (Oxford, 1924).
Berry, R. J. A., *Brain and Mind or the Nervous System of Man* (London and New York, 1928).
Bertram, G. C. L., 'The making and taking of life', *Eugenics Review*, Vol. 55, No. 3, Oct 1963, pp. 159–65.

SELECT BIBLIOGRAPHY

Besant, Annie, *Euthanasia* (London, 1875).

Blacker, C. P. *Voluntary Sterilization* (London, 1934).

—— *Eugenics in Retrospect and Prospect* (London, 1950).

Bond, C. J., *On the Meaning of Evil and Suffering* (Leicester, 1937).

Bonser, T. O., *The Right to Die* (London, 1885).

Booker, Revd Luke, *Euthanasia; Or The State of Man After Death* (London, 1822).

Bradley, F. H., 'Some remarks on punishment', *International Journal of Ethics*, Apr. 1894.

Brewer, Colin, '"Insufficient Evidence" – or a subtle shift in policy on euthanasia?', *World Medicine*, 13 Jan. 1979.

British Medical Association, *Euthanasia: Report of the Working Party to Review the British Medical Association's Guidance on Euthanasia* (London, 1988).

Bullar, Joseph, 'On the use of small doses of opium in the act of dying from phthisis', *Assoc. Med. J. London* (London, 1856).

Carrel, Alexis, *Man the Unknown* (London, 1936).

Chesterton, G. K., 'Euthanasia and murder', *American Law Review*, Vol. 8, 1937.

Church of England Board for Social Responsibility, *Decisions About Life and Death: A Problem in Modern Medicine* (London, 1966).

Church of England Board for Social Responsibility, *On Dying Well: An Anglican Contribution to the Debate on Euthanasia* (London, 1975).

Cole, Revd George, *Euthanasia, Sermons And Poems, In Memory of Departed Friends* (London, 1868).

Darwin, Charles, *The Descent of Man and Selection in Relation to Sex*, facsimile copy of the 1871 edition (Princeton, 1981).

Darwin, Leonard, *The Need for Eugenic Reform* (London, 1926).

Donne, John, *Biathanatos* (London, 1648).

Downing, A. B. (ed.), *Euthanasia and the Right to Death: The Case for Voluntary Euthanasia* (London, 1969).

Earengey, W. G., 'Voluntary euthanasia', *The Medico-legal and Criminological Review*, Vol. 8, 1940.

Ellis, Havelock, *More Essays of Love and Virtue* (London, 1931).

—— 'The Sterilisation of the Unfit', *Eugenics Review*, Vol. 1, 1909, pp. 204–6.

—— *More Essays of Love and Virtue* (London, 1931).

Exton-Smith, A. N., 'Terminal illness in the aged', *The Lancet*, 5 Aug. 1961, pp. 305–8.

Ferriar, John, *Medical Histories* (London, 1792).

Fletcher, Joseph, *Morals and Medicine* (Princeton, 1955).

Fox, Theodore, 'Purposes of medicine: the Harveian oration for 1965', *The Lancet*, 23 Oct. 1965, pp. 801–5.

French, Douglas, 'The care of cancer in practice', *The Practitioner*, Vol. 177, 1956, pp. 79–87.

Gavey, Clarence John, *The Management of the 'Hopeless' Case* (London, 1952).

Gisborne, F. A. W., *Democracy on Trial* (London, 1928).

Goddard, Charles, *Suggestions in Favour of Terminating Absolutely Hopeless Cases of Injury or Disease* (London, 1901).

Green, Peter, *The Problem of Right Conduct* (London, 1931).

Hammond, T. E., 'Euthanasia', *The Practitioner*, Vol. 132, 1934, pp. 485–94.

Haycraft, John Berry, *Darwinism and Race Progress* (London, 1895).

Hinton, J. M., 'The physical and mental distress of the dying', *Quarterly Journal of*

Medicine, New Series, Vol. 32, No. 125, Jan. 1963, pp. 1–21.

Hook, Sidney, 'Suicide', *International Journal of Ethics*, 1927.

Humphry, Derek, *Jean's Way* (London, 1978).

Inge, W. R., *Christian Ethics and Modern Problems* (London, 1930).

Keay, John, 'War and the burden of insanity', *Journal of Mental Science*, Oct. 1918, Vol. 64, No. 267, pp. 325–45.

Kennedy, Foster, 'The problem of social control of the congenitally defective: education, sterilisation, euthanasia', *American Journal of Psychiatry*, Vol. 99, 1942, pp. 13–16.

Lankester, E. R., *Degeneration: A Chapter in Darwinism* (London, 1880).

Lennox, W. G., 'Should they live? Certain economic aspects of medicine', *American Scholar*, Vol. 7, 1938, pp. 454–66.

Lorber, John, 'Results of treatment of myelomeningocele', *Developmental Medicine and Child Neurology*, Vol. 13, 1971.

Maeterlinck, M. Maurice, *Death* (London, 1911).

Mallock, W. H., 'Is life worth living?', *The Nineteenth Century*, Vol. 2, 1877, pp. 251, Vol. 3, 1878, pp. 146–68.

Maudsley, Henry, *The Physiology and Pathology of Mind* (London, 1868).

Millard, C. K., 'The Legalisation of voluntary euthanasia', *Public Health*, Vol. 45, 1931, pp. 39–47.

—— 'The case for euthanasia', *Fortnightly Review*, Dec. 1931, pp. 701–18.

—— *The Movement in Favour of Voluntary Euthanasia: An Historical Survey* (Leicester, 1936).

Moore, Charles, *A Full Inquiry into the Subject of Suicide* (London, 1790).

Munk, William, *Euthanasia: or Medical Treatment in Aid of an Easy Death* (London, 1887).

Newman, F. W., *The Bigot and the Sceptic: What is their Euthanasia?* (London, 1869).

Office of Health Economics, *Old Age* (London, 1968).

Perry-Coste, F. H., *The Ethics of Suicide* (London, 1898).

Radcliffe, J. N., 'The aesthetics of suicide', *Journal of Psychological Medicine*, Vol. 12, 1859, pp. 582–602.

Rentoul, Robert Reid, *Race Culture or Race Suicide? A Plea for the Unborn* (London, 1906).

Roberts, Harry, *Euthanasia and Other Aspects of Life and Death* (London, 1936).

Roper, A. G., *Ancient Eugenics* (Oxford, 1913).

Royal Society of Medicine, *Proceedings of the Royal Society of Medicine*, Vol. 60, Nov. 1967. 'Symposium on the cost of life.'

Russell, John, 'The ethics of suicide', *Transactions of the Medico-Legal Society*, Vol. 17, 1922, pp. 24–56.

Saleeby, C. W., 'The dysgenics of war', *Contemporary Review*, Vol. 107, 1915.

Saunby, Robert, *Medical Ethics: A Guide to Professional Conduct* (London, 1902).

Saunders Cicely, 'The problem of euthanasia', *Nursing Times*, 9 Oct. 1959, pp. 960–1.

—— 'Should a patient know?', *Nursing Times*, 16 Oct. 1959, pp. 994–5.

—— 'Control of pain in terminal cancer', *Nursing Times*, 23 Oct. 1959, pp. 1031–2.

—— 'Mental distress in the dying', *Nursing Times*, 30 Oct. 1959, pp. 1067–9.

—— 'The nursing of patients dying of cancer', *Nursing Times*, 6 Nov. 1959, pp. 1091–2.

Sorley, Charles, *The Letters of Charles Sorley* (Cambridge, 1919).

Thomson, G. P., 'An appeal to doctors', *The Lancet*, 20 Dec. 1969, p. 1353.

SELECT BIBLIOGRAPHY

Tidy, Charles, *Legal Medicine* (London, 1882).
Tollemache, Lionel, *Stones of Stumbling* (London, 1884).
Tredgold, A. F., *Mental Deficiency: Amentia* (London, 1908).
—— *Mental Deficiency: Amentia*, 4th edn (London, 1922).
—— *Mental Deficiency: Amentia*, 7th edn (London, 1947).
Tylor, Edward B., 'Primitive society', *The Contemporary Review*, Vol. 21, 1873, pp. 701–18.
Walker, J. V., 'Attitudes to death', *Gerontologia Clinica*, Vol. 10, 1968, pp. 304–8.
Ward, B. J. and Tate, P. A., 'Attitudes among NHS doctors to request for euthanasia', *British Medical Journal*, Vol. 308, 21 May 1994, pp. 1332–4.
Wells, H. G., *Anticipations* (London, 1902).
Westermarck, Edward, 'Suicide: a chapter in comparative ethics', *Sociological Review*, Vol. 1, 1908, pp. 12–33.
Westermarck, Edward, *Christianity and Morals* (London, 1939).
White, Arnold, *The Problems of a Great City* (London, 1887).
Williams, Glanville, *The Sanctity of Human Life and the Criminal Law* (London, 1958).
Williams, S. D. 'Euthanasia', *Essays of the Birmingham Speculative Club* (London, 1870).
Wilson, R. A., 'A medico-literary causerie, euthanasia', *The Practitioner*, Vol. 56, 1896, pp. 631–5.
Zachary, R. B., 'Ethical and social aspects of treatment of spina bifida', *The Lancet*, 3 Oct. 1969.

Secondary sources

Published books and articles

Ackerknecht, Erwin, 'Death in the history of medicine', *Bulletin of the History of Medicine*, Vol. 42, No. 1, 1968, pp. 19–23.
Anderson, Olive, 'Did suicide increase with industrialization in Victorian England?', *Past and Present*, Vol. 86, 1980, pp. 149–73.
—— *Suicide in Victorian and Edwardian England* (Oxford, 1987).
Bannister, R. C., 'The survival of the fittest – history or histrionics?', *Journal of the History of Ideas*, Vol. 31, July/Sep. 1970.
Barker, David, 'How to curb the fertility of the unfit: the feeble-minded in Edwardian Britain', *Oxford Review of Education*, Vol. 9, No. 3, 1983, pp. 197–211.
Barnes, J., *Ahead of his Age: Bishop Barnes of Birmingham* (London, 1979).
Bennett, Olivia, *Annie Besant* (London, 1988).
Benzenhöfer, U., 'Kindereuthanasie im Dritten Reich, Der Fall "Kind Knauer"', *Deutsches Ärzteblatt*, 95, Heft 19, 8 Mai 1998, pp. 954–5.
Berrios, G. and Freeman, H. (eds), *150 Years of British Psychiatry* (London, 1991).
Bliss, Michael, *William Osler: A Life in Medicine* (Oxford, 1999).
Bowler, Peter, *Charles Darwin: The Man and his Influence* (Oxford, 1990, reprinted Cambridge, 1996).
—— *The Fontana History of the Environmental Sciences* (London, 1992).
Briant, Keith, *Marie Stopes: A Biography* (London, 1962).
Brookes, Barbara, *Abortion in Britain 1900–1967* (London, 1988).

Bryder, Lynda, *Below the Magic Mountain* (Oxford, 1989).

Burleigh, Michael, '"Euthanasia" in the Third Reich: some recent literature', *Social History of Medicine*, Vol. 4, 1991, pp. 317–28.

—— *Death and Deliverance: 'Euthanasia' In Germany 1900–1945* (Cambridge, 1994).

—— *Ethics and Extermination: Reflections on Nazi Genocide* (Cambridge, 1997).

Burleigh, Michael and Wippermann, Wolfgang, *The Racial State: Germany 1933–1945* (Cambridge, 1991)

Burnett, John, *Early Greek Philosophy* (London, 1892).

Bynum, W. F., Porter, R., and Shepherd, M. (eds), *The Anatomy of Madness*, 3 vols. (London, 1985–88).

Bynum, W. F. and Porter Roy (eds), *The Companion Encyclopedia of the History of Medicine* (London, 1993).

Carneiro, Robert (ed.), *Selections from Herbert Spencer's Principles of Sociology* (Chicago, 1967).

Chadwick, Owen, *The Victorian Church: Part 2* (London, 1970).

—— *The Secularisation of the European Mind in the Nineteenth Century* (Cambridge 1975, reprinted 1995).

Clarke, David, 'Someone to watch over me', *Nursing Times*, Vol. 93, No. 34, 20 Aug. 1997.

Collini, Stephan, *Public Moralists: Political Thought and Intellectual Life in Britain 1850–1930* (Oxford, 1991).

Cowan, R. S., 'Nature and nurture: the interplay of biology and politics in the thought of Francis Galton', *Studies in the History of Biology*, Vol. 1, 1977, pp. 133–208.

David, Hugh, *On Queer Street: A Social History of Homosexuality 1895–1995* (London, 1997).

Davies, Christie, *Permissive Britain. Social Change in the Sixties and Seventies* (London, 1975).

Dawtry, Frank, 'The abolition of the death penalty in Britain', *British Journal of Criminology*, Vol. 6, Apr 1966, pp. 183–92.

Du Boulay, Shirley, *Cicely Saunders: Founder of the Modern Hospice Movement* (London, 1984).

Dworkin, Ronald, *Life's Dominion: An Argument about Abortion and Euthanasia* (London, 1993).

Edelstein, Ludwig, 'The Hippocratic Oath', *Supplement to the Bulletin of the History of Medicine*, No. 1 (Baltimore, 1943).

Emanuel, Ezekiel, J. 'The history of euthanasia debates in the United States and Britain', *Annals of Internal Medicine*, Vol. 121, No. 10, Nov 1994.

—— *The Ends of Human Life: Medical Ethics in a Liberal Polity* (Cambridge, Massachusetts, 1991).

Farrell, L. A., *The Origins and Growth of the English Eugenics Movement 1865–1925* (New York, 1985).

Fedden, H. R., *Suicide: A Social and Historical Study* (London, 1938).

Fisher, Trevor, 'Permissiveness and the politics of morality', *Contemporary Record*, Vol. 7, No. 1, Summer 1993, pp. 149–65.

Folb, P. I., *The Thalidomide Disaster and its Impact on Modern Medicine* (Cape Town, 1977).

Foot, Michael, *H. G. The History of Mr Wells* (London, 1995).

Forrest, D. W., *Francis Galton: The Life and Work of a Victorian Genius* (New York, 1974).

SELECT BIBLIOGRAPHY

Foucault, Michel, *Madness and Civilization* (London, 1967).

Freeden, Michael, 'Eugenics and progressive thought: a study in ideological affinity', *Historical Journal*, Vol. 22, 1979, pp. 645–71.

Friedlander, Henry, *The Origins of Nazi Genocide: From Euthanasia To The Final Solution* (London, 1995).

Fussell, Paul, *The Great War and Modern Memory* (Oxford, 1975).

Fye, W. Bruce, 'Active euthanasia: an historical survey of its conceptional origins and introduction into medical thought', *Bulletin of the History of Medicine* (Baltimore, 1968) pp. 493–502.

Gilley, Sheridan and Sheils, W. J. (eds), *A History of Religion in Britain* (Oxford, 1994).

Gillon, Ranaan, 'Suicide and voluntary euthanasia: historical perspectives', in Downing, A. B. (ed.), *Euthanasia and the Right to Die* (London, 1969).

Glover, Jonathan, *Causing Death and Saving Lives* (London, [1977] 1990).

Gould, Stephen Jay, *The Mismeasure of Man* (London, 1981).

Gourevitch, Danielle, 'Suicide among the sick in classical antiquity', *Bulletin of the History of Medicine*, No. 43 (Baltimore, 1969).

Grosskarth, P., *Havelock Ellis* (London, 1980).

Halliday, R. J., 'Social Darwinism: a definition', *Victorian Studies*, Vol. 14, 1971.

Harris, Jose, *Private Lives Public Spirit: Britain 1870–1914* (Oxford, [1993] 1994).

Harrison, Brian, *Drink and the Victorians* (London, 1971).

Hawkins, Mike, *Social Darwinism in European and American Thought 1860–1945* (Cambridge, 1997).

Helme, Tim, 'The Voluntary Euthanasia (Legalisation) Bill (1936) revisited', *Journal of Medical Ethics*, Vol. 17, 1991, pp. 25–9.

Hilton, Boyd, *Age of Atonement* (Oxford, 1988).

Holmes, S. J., *A Bibliography of Eugenics* (Berkeley, 1924).

Houlbrook, Ralph (ed.), *Death Ritual and Bereavement* (London, 1989).

Hume, David, 'Of suicide', published posthumously in 1784 and reprinted from the *The Philosophical Works of David Hume*, (eds), Green, T. H. and Gosse T. H. (London, 1874–75) in Singer, Peter (ed.), *Applied Ethics* (Oxford, 1986), pp. 19–27.

Jackson, Mark, *New-born Child Murder: Women, Illegitimacy and the Courts in Eighteenth-Century England* (Manchester, 1996).

—— *The Borderland of Imbecility: Medicine, Society and the Fabrication of the Feeble-mind in Later Victorian and Edwardian England* (Manchester, 2000).

Jalland, Pat, *Death in the Victorian Family* (Oxford, 1996).

Jones, Greta, *Social Darwinism in English Thought* (Brighton, 1980).

—— 'Eugenics and social policy between the wars', *Historical Journal*, Vol. 25, 1982, pp. 717–28.

—— *Social Hygiene in Twentieth-Century Britain* (London, 1986).

Karlen, Arno, *Plague's Progress* (London, 1995).

Kennedy, Ian, 'The legal effect of requests by the terminally ill and aged not to receive further treatment from doctors', *Criminal Law Review*, 1976, pp. 217–32.

Kent, Christopher, 'Higher journalism and the mid-Victorian clerisy', *Victorian Studies*, Vol. 13, 1969, pp. 181–98.

Keown, J., *Abortion, Doctors, and the Law: Some Aspects of the Legal Regulation of Abortion in England from 1803 to 1982* (Cambridge, 1988).

Kevles, Daniel, *In the Name of Eugenics: Genetics and the Uses of Human Heredity* (New York, 1985).

Kitcher, Philip, *The Lives to Come: The Genetic Revolution and Human Possibilities* (London, 1996).

Kohl, Marvin (ed.), *Beneficent Euthanasia* (New York, 1975).

Kühl, Stefan, *The Nazi Connection: Eugenics, American Racism, and German National Socialism* (Oxford, 1994).

Kuhse, Helga and Singer, Peter, *Should the Baby Live?* (Oxford, 1985).

Lawrence, Christopher, *Medicine in the Making of Modern Britain 1700–1920* (London, 1994).

Lomax, E., 'The uses and abuses of opiates in nineteenth century England', *Bulletin of the History of Medicine*, Vol. 47, 1973, pp. 167–76.

MacDonald, Michael, and Murphy, Terence, *Sleepless Souls: Suicide in Early Modern England* (Oxford, 1990).

Macnicol, John, 'Eugenics and the campaign for voluntary sterilisation in Britain between the wars', *Social History of Medicine*, Vol. 2, No. 2, August 1989.

Macquitty, B., *Battle for Oblivion: The Discovery of Anaesthesia* (London, 1969).

Mackenzie, Donald, *Statistics in Britain 1865–1910. The Social Construction of Scientific Knowledge* (Edinburgh, 1981).

Marwick, Arthur, *British Society Since 1945* (Harmondsworth, 1982).

—— *The Sixties* (Oxford, 1998).

Maude, A., *The Life Of Marie Stopes* (London, 1933).

Mazumdar, Pauline, *Eugenics, Human Genetics, and Human Failings* (London, 1992).

McCabe, Joseph, *A Biographical Dictionary of Modern Rationalists* (London, 1920).

McConnaughey, G., 'Social Darwinism', *Osiris*, Vol. 9, 1950.

McKeown, Thomas, *Medicine in Modern Society: Medical Planning Based on Evaluation of Medical Achievement* (London, 1965).

McKibbin, Ross, *Classes and Cultures: England 1918–1951* (Oxford, 1998).

McNeil, William, *Plagues and Peoples* (Oxford, 1977).

Noakes, Jeremy and Geoffrey, Pridham (eds), *Nazism 1919–1945, Vol. 3, Foreign Policy, War and Racial Extermination: A Documentary Reader* (Exeter, [1988] 1991)

Newsome, David, *The Victorian World Picture* (London, 1997).

Paul, D., 'Eugenics and the left', *Journal of the History of Ideas*, Vol. 45, 1984, pp. 561–90.

Peel, J. D. Y., *Herbert Spencer, the Evolution of a Sociologist* (London, 1971).

—— (ed.), *Herbert Spencer On Social Evolution Selected Writings* (Chicago, 1972).

Pernick, Martin, *A Calculus of Suffering* (New York, 1986).

—— *The Black Stork: Eugenics and the death of Defective Babies in American Medicine and Motion Pictures Since 1915* (New York, Oxford, 1996).

Pick, Daniel, *Faces of Degeneration: A European Disorder, c. 1848–1918* (Cambridge, 1989).

Porter, Dorothy, '"Enemies of the Race": biologism, environmentalism, and public health in Edwardian England', *Victorian Studies*, Vol. 34, Winter 1991, pp. 159–78.

Porter, Roy and Hall, Lesley, *The Facts of Life: The Creation of Sexual Knowledge in Britain, 1650–1950* (London, 1995).

Porter, Roy, *The Greatest Benefit to Mankind: A Medical History of Humanity from Antiquity to the Present* (London, 1997).

SELECT BIBLIOGRAPHY

—— *The Cambridge Illustrated History of Medicine* (Cambridge, 1996)

Proctor, Robert, *Racial Hygiene. Medicine Under the Nazis* (Cambridge, Massachusetts, 1988).

Quine, Maria Sophia, *Population Politics in Twentieth-Century Europe* (London, 1996).

Raine, Craig, *History: The Home Movie* (London, 1994).

Rey, Roselyne, *The History of Pain* (Paris, 1993, Cambridge, Massachusetts, 1998).

Robbins, William, *The Newman Brothers: An Essay in Comparative Intellectual Biography* (London, 1966).

Rogers, James A., 'Darwinism and social Darwinism', *Journal of the History of Ideas*, Vol. 33, May/June 1972.

Sandbach, F. H., *The Stoics* (London [1975] 1994).

Schreiber, Bernard, *The Men Behind Hitler* (London, c. 1972).

Scull, Andrew, *Social Order/Mental Disorder: Anglo-American Psychiatry in Historical Perspective* (London, 1989).

Searle, G. R., *The Quest for National Efficiency* (Oxford, 1971).

—— *Eugenics and Politics, 1900–1914* (Leyden, 1976)

—— 'Eugenics and Politics in Britain in the 1930s', *Annals of Science*, Vol. 36, 1979, pp. 159–69.

Sereny, Gitta, *Into That Darkness: From Mercy Killing to Mass Murder* (London, 1995).

Shorter, Edward, *A History of Psychiatry* (New York, 1997).

Singer, Peter, *Practical Ethics* (Cambridge, 1993).

—— *Rethinking Life and Death* (Oxford, 1995).

Singer, Peter (ed.), *A Companion to Ethics* (Oxford, 1995).

Smith, W. D. A., *Under the Influence: 200 Years of Nitrous Oxide and Oxygen* (London, 1982).

Soloway, Richard, *Birth Control and the Population Question in England, 1877–1930* (London, 1986).

—— *Demography and Degeneration: Eugenics and the Declining Birthrate in Twentieth-Century Britain* (London, 1990).

Spencer, Colin, *The Heretic's Feast: A History of Vegetarianism* (London, 1993).

Sprott, S. E., *The English Debate on Suicide from Donne to Hume* (Illinois, 1961).

Stevenson, John, *British Society 1914–45* (London [1984] 1990).

Stewart, Herbert, 'Euthanasia', *International Journal of Ethics*, 1918.

Szreter, Simon, 'The importance of social intervention in Britain's mortality decline, c. 1850–1914: a reinterpretation of the role of public health', *Social History of Medicine*, Vol. 1, 1988, pp. 1–38.

Thomson, Mathew, 'Sterilisation, segregation, and community care: ideology and the problem of mental deficiency in inter-war Britain', *History of Psychiatry*, Vol. 3, 1992, pp. 473–98.

—— *The Problem of Mental Deficiency: Eugenics, Democracy, and Social Policy in Britain c. 1870–1959* (Oxford, 1998).

Turner, Frank, *The Greek Heritage in Victorian Britain* (London, 1981).

Van Der Sluis, I., 'The movement for euthanasia 1875–1975', *Janus*, Vol. 66, pp. 131–72.

Vidler, Alec, *The Church in an Age of Revolution* (London, 1961).

Watson, Francis, 'The death of George V', *History Today*, Vol. 36, 1986.

Webster, Charles, *The Health Services Since the War Vol. 2: Government and Health*

Care The National Health Service 1958–1979 (London, 1996).

Weindling, Paul, *Health Race and German Politics Between National Unification and Nazism 1870–1945* (Cambridge, 1989).

Weingart, Peter, 'Eugenic utopias – blueprints for the rationalization of human evolution', *Sociology of the Sciences*, 1984, pp. 173–87.

Welshman, John, 'Eugenics and public health in Britain, 1900–40: scenes from provincial life', *Urban History*, May 1997.

Wilkinson, Alan, *The Church of England and the First World War* (London, [1978] 1996).

Wright, David and Digby, Anne, (eds), *From Idiocy to Mental Deficiency: Historical Perspectives on People with Learning Disabilities* (London, 1996).

Unpublished theses

Buchanan, E. E., 'Aspects of the life and times of Dr Charles Killick Millard, 1901–1934', University of Leicester MA thesis, 1995

Condliffe, Robin, 'Merciful release? A history of the British Voluntary Euthanasia Movement', B.Sc. thesis, University of London, 1994–95.

Gildea, Maureen, 'Euthanasia: A review of the American literature', senior thesis, Harvard University, 1983.

Morrice, A. A. G., 'Honour and interests: Medical ethics in Britain, and the work of the British Medical Association's Central Ethical Committee, 1902–1939', MD thesis, University of London, 1999.

Index